Nutrition
and
Drugs

CURRENT CONCEPTS IN NUTRITION

Myron Winick, Editor

Institute of Human Nutrition
Columbia University College of Physicians and Surgeons

Nutrition and Drugs

Edited by

MYRON WINICK

Institute of Human Nutrition
Columbia University College of
Physicians and Surgeons

A WILEY-INTERSCIENCE PUBLICATION
JOHN WILEY & SONS
New York • Chichester • Brisbane • Toronto • Singapore

Library of Congress Cataloging in Publication Data:

Main entry under title:

Nutrition and drugs.

  (Current concepts in nutrition ; v. 12)
  "A Wiley-Interscience Publication."
  Includes index.
  1. Drug-nutrient interactions. I. Winick, Myron.
II. Series. [DNLM: 1. Diet therapy. 2. Drug interactions. 3. Drug therapy. 4. Nutrition—Drug effects.
5. Nutrition disorders—Chemically induced. W1 CU788AS
v. 12 / QU 4 N976]

RM302.4.N87 1983   615'.7045   83-1187
ISBN 0-471-89210-6

Printed in the United States of America
10 9 8 7 6 5 4 3 2 1

Preface

This volume discusses the interaction of diet and drugs. In our society the consumption of drugs has reached unprecedented levels. Advances in medicine and the use of pharmacological agents for specific treatment of disease account for the use of some drugs. Others are used by the medical profession to control troublesome symptoms of certain illnesses. Still others, the vast majority, are sold "over the counter" and are used by the general public for everything from pain control to prevention of anxiety. Aside from their specific actions most drugs have side effects some of which interfere with the metabolism of certain nutrients. In this volume we will discuss some of the most important of these drugs and the mechanisms by which they impair the transport, absorption, and metabolism of certain important nutrients.

Drugs have also become a part of our food supply. Two such drugs, alcohol and caffeine, are consumed in very large quantities. These drugs are potent pharmacologic agents and their abuse may lead to serious health problems. The metabolism of alcohol is discussed in detail by Charles Lieber. In this chapter the mechanisms by which alcohol produces its direct effects are carefully described. The indirect effects of alcohol consumption, particularly those effects which alter the metabolism of important nutrients, are also discussed. Caffeine is examined by Dr. Sanford Miller in a chapter on early development and the potential dangers of caffeine during pregnancy and childhood.

Certain nutrients in high doses or analogs of these nutrients have potent physiologic and pharmacologic effects. Both vitamin D and vitamin A fall into this category. Analogs of the dihydroxy form of vitamin D have been used with some success in the treatment of osteoporosis, and the use of vitamin A analogs is being examined in skin diseases. The present state of the art in using these two analogs is examined.

In the treatment of certain diseases a combination of drugs and nutritional therapy is employed. Obesity is one of these conditions. The latest research on newer drugs that suppress appetite and on the efficacy of such drugs in the treatment of obesity is considered. Hypertension, diabetes, and atherosclerosis are all treated with drugs and diet. The last part of this book considers these three diseases and the interaction of diet and drugs in their control.

This volume is not designed to cover the interaction of all drugs with nutrients derived from our diet. Instead certain examples have been chosen which illustrate important general principles for physicians and nutritionists to consider in the management of their patients.

MYRON WINICK

New York, New York
April 1983

Contents

Nutrition
and
Drugs

1

Drug–Vitamin B$_6$ Interaction

HEMMIGE N. BHAGAVAN, Ph.D. and
MYRON BRIN, Ph.D.

Hoffman-La Roche Inc., Nutley, New Jersey

The subject of drug-nutrient interactions is an important one which has practical implications. An excellent book on the subject has been written by Roe (1). In a more recent article Brin and Roe (2) discuss the general problem of drug-nutrient and pollutant-nutrient interactions and provide a rationale for the concept of marginal nutritional deficiencies.

Several classes of drugs are known to interfere with vitamin B$_6$ metabolism; examples of this interaction are shown in Table 1. Among these drugs are antituberculous, anti-Parkinson, anti-Wilson, and antifertility (oral contraceptives) agents. For the purposes of this discussion, alcohol is also considered a drug.

**Table 1. Vitamin B$_6$ and
Drug Interactions**

Alcohol
Antituberculous drugs (INH; cycloserine)
Anti-Parkinson drugs (L-DOPA)
Anti-Wilson drugs (D-penicillamine)
Oral contraceptives

VITAMIN B$_6$ METABOLISM

The metabolic interconversions of vitamin B$_6$ are outlined in Figure 1. Pyridoxal-5'-phosphate (PLP) is the key coenzyme which can arise by way of either pyridoxal (PAL) or pyridoxine-5'-phosphate. PLP plays an

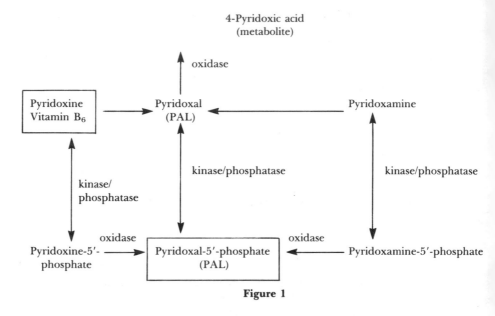

Figure 1

important coenzymatic role in numerous pathways in amino acid metabolism. The typical reactions catalyzed by PLP are represented in Table 2.

PLP and PAL are very reactive compounds which can readily complex with a variety of compounds bearing an amino group to form Schiff-type bases. This results in the functional inactivation of both PLP and the drug in question, and this inactivation underlies one important mechanism in the interaction between vitamin B$_6$ and drugs.

Table 2.   Typical Reaction Types Catalyzed by PLP

1. Transamination
2. Decarboxylation
3. Amine oxidation
4. Aldol reaction
5. Cleavage reaction
6. Dehydration
7. Desulfhydration
8. Synthesis
9. Racemization

Table 3. Recommended Dietary Allowance (1980) Vitamin B₆ (mg/day)

Subjects	Age (Yr)	Allowance
Infants	0–1	0.3–0.6
Children	1–3	0.9
	4–6	1.3
	7–10	1.6
Males	11–18	1.8–2.0
	19–51+	2.2
Females	11–14	1.8
	15–51+	2.0
Pregnant		+0.6
Lactating		+0.5

RECOMMENDED DIETARY ALLOWANCE

Before discussing the interaction between vitamin B₆ and various types of drugs, let us consider the latest (1980) recommended dietary allowances (RDA) for vitamin B₆ (3). The requirements are shown in Table 3 with age and sex breakdown. For adults over 19 years (females and males) they are 2.0 mg and 2.2 mg, respectively, a day, and these are for normal healthy Americans. The vitamin B₆ needs of patients during drug therapy will be discussed in the following paragraphs, and the recommended dosages usually are generally well above the RDA.

VITAMIN B₆ MARGINAL DEFICIENCY

Generally, the vitamin B₆ inadequacy that may occur as a consequence of drug or environmental chemical interaction results in a marginal deficiency, and in some cases clinical signs may be manifested. Presented in Table 4 is a sequence of events in the development of vitamin deficiency (4). Stages 1 and 2 can be revealed only by biochemical evaluation, while in stage 3 there are signs and symptoms which are nonspecific. Only if the depletion reaches stages 4 and 5 can the problem be accurately attributed to a particular vitamin deficiency. Although overt clinical effects can be seen only toward the end of the depletion sequence, the biochemical studies show a smooth transition of reduced function throughout the five stages. Relating the biochemical state to the clinical findings permits one to appreciate the broad meaning of nutritional in-

Table 4.   Stages in the Development of Vitamin Deficiency

Stage	Event
1. Preliminary	Inadequate availability (diet, malabsorption, abnormal metabolism, etc.)
2. Biochemical	Reduced tissue content and decreased urinary excretion; reduced enzyme and coenzyme activity
3. Physiological and behavioral	Reduced appetite and weight loss; insomnia; irritability; general malaise
4. Clinical	Classical deficiency symptoms
5. Terminal	Tissue pathology; death if condition not promptly corrected

adequacy. It is therefore apparent that the absence of clinical signs does not necessarily imply normal function.

Alcohol

It is known that chronic alcoholics suffer from malnutrition that has a complex etiology. The malnutrition can be either primary or secondary as indicated in Table 5. The primary problem may be due to insufficient nutrient intake or to decreased appetite related to liver-gastrointestinal problems. In secondary malnutrition, the impaired nutrient utilization may be related to any of the following factors: alcohol-induced gastrointestinal damage, deficiency-induced malabsorption, impaired function. With respect to vitamin B$_6$, data show that alcohol ingestion decreases plasma PLP values, thus indicating an adverse effect on vitamin B$_6$ me-

Table 5.   Alcohol–Nutrient Interaction

Primary malnutrition
   Insufficient intake
   Impaired appetite
     (GI–liver disorders)

Secondary malnutrition
   Impaired utilization
     GI damage (alcohol-induced)
     Malabsorption (deficiency-induced)
     Impaired function (viz., coenzyme)

Table 6. Vitamin and Mineral Depletion in Alcoholism

	Vitamins	Minerals
Vitamin A	Thiamine	Magnesium
Vitamin D	Riboflavin	Calcium
	Niacin	Zinc
	Pyridoxine	Iron
	Folic acid	
	Vitamin B$_{12}$	
	Ascorbic acid	

tabolism and function. The sideroblastic anemia seen in alcoholics has been attributed to a decreased synthesis of PLP from pyridoxine (5). More recent data with experimental animals also support impairment of PLP synthesis (6). According to Veitch et al. (7), there is an increased catabolism of PLP (increased phosphatase activity) in chronic alcoholism. Both processes can lead to a decrease in the functional vitamin B$_6$ status. As shown in Table 6, the status of a number of other vitamins and minerals is also impaired in alcoholism. The neurological problems associated with alcoholism may be attributable, in part, to impaired functional status not only of vitamin B$_6$, but also of other vitamins, such as vitamin B$_1$ (1).

Hydrazines

A variety of drugs belong to the family of hydrazines, as shown in Table 7. Among these are antidepressants, antihypertensives, and antituberculous drugs. Isonicotinylhydrazide, commonly known as INH, belongs to the last group, and has been widely investigated with

Table 7. Hydrazine Derivatives

Antidepressants	Iproniazid
	Nialamid (Niamid)
	Isocarboxazid (Marplan)
MAO inhibitors	Phenalzine (Nardil)
Antituberculous agents	Isonicotinylhydrazide (INH)
Antihypertensive agents	Hydralazine (Apresoline)
Anticarcinogenic agents	Procarbazine (Natulan)

Table 8.   INH (Isonicotinylhydrazide)

Side effects
  Behavioral changes
    Hyperkinesis; irritability; sleep problems
  Mental changes
    Psychosis; lowered consciousness level
  Neurological changes
    Peripheral neuropathy; convulsions
Excellent response to vitamin B$_6$ therapy (dose-dependent)

particular reference to its interaction with vitamin B$_6$. In theory, any hydrazine derivative is a potential antivitamin B$_6$ compound by virtue of its ability to form a hydrazone with PAL or PLP. In this context, it is interesting to note that the effects on the central nervous system observed in workers exposed to the hydrazine type of rocket fuel have been attributed to its antagonism of vitamin B$_6$ (1).

INH is extensively used in the treatment of tuberculosis. The side effects of INH are listed in Table 8, and include both behavioral and neurological changes. The symptoms can be reversed by adequate vitamin B$_6$ therapy without interfering with the clinical efficacy of INH. There are several instances where either intentional (suicide) or accidental INH overdosing resulted in convulsions or other symptoms. In such cases the therapy calls for dose-dependent administration of vitamin B$_6$, often by the intravenous route. It is interesting to note that no adverse effects of vitamin B$_6$ have been noticed following intravenous administration of very high doses (70–357 mg/kg body weight) of the vitamin (8).

The mechanisms involved in the interaction between vitamin B$_6$ and INH are given in Table 9. In addition to forming hydrazone with PLP, INH also acts as a competitive inhibitor of certain PLP-enzymes. The sei-

Table 9.   Mechanism: Vitamin B$_6$–INH Interaction

1. INH + PAL/PLP → Hydrazone → urinary excretion
2. Competitive inhibition: PLP enzymes

$$\text{INH}$$
$$\downarrow$$

3. Brain glutamate decarboxylase $\rightarrow$ GABA
4. Seizure activity → lactate (lactic acidosis)

$$\text{NAD} \downarrow \leftarrow \text{INH}$$
$$\text{pyruvate}$$

zure activity due to INH toxicity has been attributed to the inhibition of brain glutamate decarboxylase, a PLP-dependent enzyme, resulting in the decreased availability of the inhibitory neurotransmitter γ-aminobutyric acid (GABA).

A unique side effect of INH, by way of unmasking a vitamin B$_6$ dependency disorder, has been described in the literature. There are individuals who are otherwise normal, but are genetically predisposed to a vitamin B$_6$ dependency problem. In one such case, a girl aged 3 showed behavioral deterioration with hyperkinesis. Treatment with vitamin B$_6$ (100–400 mg/day) led to complete remission, and the patient was then placed on maintenance therapy (300–400 mg/day). Even short-term disruption resulted in hyperkinesis and other behavioral problems (9).

Cycloserine

Cycloserine is another drug that has been used extensively and effectively in the treatment of tuberculosis, especially in cases resistant to INH-para-aminosalicylic acid-streptomycin therapy. The side effects are primarily confined to the central nervous system, and involve neurological and neuropsychiatric changes such as sedation, consciousness lowering, and seizure activity (Table 10). The symptoms have been attributed to interference with vitamin B$_6$ metabolism, and cycloserine is now recognized as a vitamin B$_6$ antagonist. The mechanism involves the formation of a Schiff base with PLP which then leads to the production of an oxime. These processes result in an inactivation of PLP. The effects of cycloserine on the central nervous system can usually be reversed by administration of large doses of vitamin B$_6$ (greater than 50 mg/day) along with the drug (10).

Table 10. Cycloserine

Side effects
   Neurological/neuropsychiatric changes
      Consciousness lowering
      Sedation
      Convulsions
   Mechanism
      Cycloserine + PLP → Schiff's base → Oxime
      (hydroxylamine derivative)
Clinical response to vitamin B$_6$ therapy (> 50 mg/day)

L-DOPA

The impairment in the dopamine neurotransmitter system in the nigraneostriatal regions of the brain has been recognized as the primary lesion in Parkinsonian patients. Exogenous dopamine is ineffective in normalizing the very low levels in critical regions of the brain because dopamine is unable to cross the blood-brain barrier. However, its precursor L-3,4-dihydroxyphenylalanine (L-DOPA) can, and presumably sufficient dopamine is formed within the brain to alleviate the symptoms of Parkinson's disease (11, 12).

L-DOPA has been in use since the sixties for treating Parkinson's patients and has now become the standard therapy for the disease. However, there are certain important side effects of the treatment, which include both neurological and behavioral problems (Table 11). These appear to be related to a vitamin B$_6$ insufficiency situation due to an interaction between L-DOPA and PLP. Although vitamin B$_6$ is essential for L-DOPA decarboxylase function, extra amounts of the vitamin in Parkinson's patients on L-DOPA alone have been found to reduce its clinical efficacy. A good deal of work has been done on the interaction between L-DOPA and vitamin B$_6$. L-DOPA can form a Schiff base with PLP, forming a tetrahydroquinoline derivative which has been reported to be inhibitory to L-DOPA decarboxylase. Another effect of L-DOPA is its possible inhibition of pyridoxal kinase, the enzyme that converts PAL to PLP.

In recent years, peripheral decarboxylase inhibitors such as carbidopa have become available. These drugs have facilitated greater delivery of L-DOPA to the brain at much lower doses. Furthermore, the clinical efficacy of the two combined drugs is not affected by vitamin B$_6$.

Table 11.   L-DOPA

Side effects
  Neurological
  Behavioral
    Anger (depressed patients)
    Mania/hypomania (manic-depressive patients)

Chronic L-DOPA → adaptive alteration in the decarboxylase system with increased ability to synthesize PLP; this explains progressive loss of L-DOPA effect

---

Table 12.   D-Penicillamine

Side effects
    Sensory neuropathy
    Motor neuropathy
    Epileptic seizures
Mechanism
    Formation of thiazolidine derivative with PLP
Clinical response to vitamin B$_6$ therapy (50 mg/day)

Penicillamine

Penicillamine is a metal-chelating agent, and because of this property, it has been in use for over two decades for the treatment of Wilson's disease (hepatolenticular degeneration) to reduce the copper load in the patients (13). It has also been used in cystinuria to prevent the formation of urinary cystine stones by facilitating the excretion of cystine as a soluble, mixed disulfide (14). The side effects of D-penicillamine therapy are mostly neurological. They include sensory and motor neuropathies and epileptic seizures (Table 12). Data from both animal studies and clinical trials indicate that D-penicillamine interferes with vitamin B$_6$ metabolism, and the symptoms seen in patients treated with D-penicillamine are likely to be due to a vitamin B$_6$ insufficiency state. It has been known for some time that D-penicillamine and PLP can combine to form a thiazolidine derivative, thus inactivating PLP (15), and this appears to be the mechanism under in vivo conditions. Nevertheless, the side effects of D-penicillamine therapy can be reversed by vitamin B$_6$ supplementation, and it has been suggested that routine D-penicillamine therapy should include supplementation with vitamin B$_6$.

Oral Contraceptives

Oral contraceptives are being used by millions of women, and several problems, particularly those related to vitamins, have been recognized for some time (Table 13). Among the biochemical changes found in oral contraceptive users (and also in pregnant women) is an abnormal tryptophan metabolism by way of increased activity of the kynurenine pathway (16, 17). Vitamin B$_6$ is involved in the metabolism of tryptophan, and there is evidence to indicate a decreased vitamin B$_6$ status in users of oral contraceptives. Previous data show that large amounts of vitamin

Table 13.   Oral Contraceptives

Side effects
  Mental symptoms
    Depression: mood changes
  Impaired glucose tolerance
  Abnormal tryptophan metabolism
  Decreased plasma vitamins B$_2$, B$_6$, B$_{12}$, C, and folate
Clinical response to vitamin B$_6$ therapy

B$_6$ (20–40 mg daily) can largely correct the abnormality in tryptophan metabolism and other associated disorders in women using these agents. (17, 18).

Mental symptoms often associated with the use of oral contraceptives include mood changes, and particularly depression. These changes are attributed to a decreased availability of tryptophan for the synthesis of the neurotransmitter serotonin due to increased metabolism by way of the kynurenine pathway (Figure 2). This is caused by the stimulation of the enzyme tryptophan 2,3-dioxygenase (pyrrolase) by steroid hormones. There is also evidence to indicate that the steroid hormones can compete with PLP for binding with apoenzymes (19).

Because of the reported side effects of oral contraceptives, the potency of the component steroid hormone (estrogen) has now been reduced (from 50 µg to 35 µg). Based on more recent reports, it has been suggested that the daily intake of vitamin B$_6$ be at least 5 mg in oral contraceptive users (20).

A study of the long-term effects of oral contraceptive use on the vitamin B$_6$ status of women who later become pregnant has recently been made by Kirksey and her associates (21). The data suggest that 5–10 mg of vitamin B$_6$ are needed to maintain plasma levels of women who were not users of these agents, whereas greater than 15 mg are required by women who were long-term oral contraceptive users.

Amphetamines

An interesting observation has recently been made on an interaction between vitamin B$_6$ and amphetamines (22). An 8-year-old boy with persistent unilateral headache was treated with Dexedrine. However, the following adverse effects were observed during therapy: compulsive rituals, tics (head and diaphragm), emotional lability, and signs of regression (including separation anxiety). A problem with vitamin B$_6$ defi-

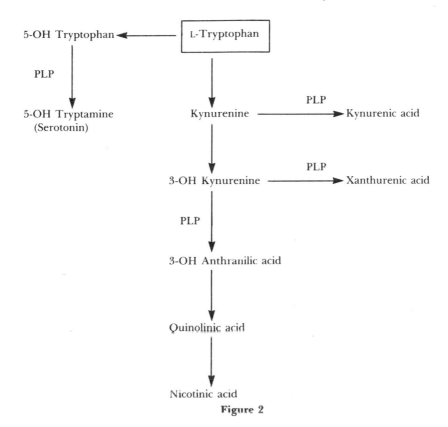

Figure 2

ciency was suspected and hence vitamin B_6 treatment was instituted (10 mg/kg) which resulted in an excellent clinical response. Although the mechanism of the interrelationship is not clear, this is yet another example of drug–vitamin B_6 interaction.

SUMMARY AND CONCLUSIONS

In conclusion, there are several drug types that can interfere with vitamin B_6 metabolism. In most cases, the interaction involves a complex formation between the drug (or a derivative) and the reactive coenzyme PLP, resulting in a Schiff base. Such an interaction leads to an inactivation of PLP (and also of the drug). Other types of interaction involve (a) stimulation of vitamin B_6-dependent pathways and (b) competition with PLP for the binding site on the enzyme. Examples of the above are the steroid hormones (oral contraceptives).

In most instances, overt symptoms of vitamin B$_6$ deficiency due to chronic ingestion of these drugs are observed, and neurological problems seem to be rather frequent. Because of the reactive nature of the coenzyme PLP and the ease with which it can interact with drugs, subclinical (marginal) vitamin B$_6$ deficiency should be suspected in the absence of overt clinical signs. Once the vitamin B$_6$ problem has been identified, the condition can usually be treated by judicious use of large doses of vitamin B$_6$ without compromising the clinical efficacy of the drug.

REFERENCES

1. D. A. Roe, *Drug-induced Nutritional Deficiencies*, Avi Publishing Co., Westport, CT, 1976.

2. M. Brin and D. Roe, *J. Fl. Med. Assoc.* **66,** 424 (1979).

3. *Recommended Dietary Allowances*, Food and Nutrition Board, National Academy of Sciences, Washington, D.C. (1980).

4. M. Brin, *J. Am. Med. Assoc.,* **187,** 762 (1964).

5. J. D. Hines, *J. Lab Clin. Med.,* **74,** 882, (1969).

6. T. H. Parker, J. P. Marshall, II, R. K. Roberts, S. Wang, E. R. Schiff, G. R. Wilkinson, and R. Schenker, *Am. J. Clin. Nutr.,* **32,** 1246 (1979).

7. R. L. Veitch, L. Lumeng, and T.-K. Li, *J. Clin. Invest.,* **55,** 1026 (1975).

8. S. Wason, P. G. Lacouture, and F. H. Lovejoy, Jr., *J. Am. Med. Assoc.,* **246,** 1102 (1981).

9. A. Brenner and R. A. Wapnir, *Am. J. Dis. Child.,* **132,** 773 (1978).

10. P. Holtz and D. Palm, *Pharmacol. Rev.,* **16,** 113 (1964).

11. K. F. Gey and A. Pletscher, *Biochem. J.,* **92,** 300 (1964).

12. G. C. Cotzias, *J. Am. Med. Assoc.,* **218,** 1903 (1971).

13. J. M. Walshe, *Am. J. Med.,* **21,** 487 (1956).

14. J. C. Crawhall and R. W. E. Watts, *Am. J. Med.,* **45,** 736 (1968).

15. D. Heyl, S. A. Harris, and K. Folkers, *J. Am. Chem. Soc.,* **70,** 3429 (1948).

16. D. P. Rose and I. P. Braidman, *Am. J. Clin. Nutr.,* **24,** 673 (1971).

17. M. Brin, *Am. J. Clin. Nutr.,* **24,** 699 (1971).

18. D. P. Rose, R. Strong, P. W. Adams, and P. E. Harding, *Clin. Sci.,* **42,** 465 (1972).

19. M. Mason, J. Ford, and H. L. C. Wu, *Ann. N.Y. Acad. Sci.,* **166,** 170 (1969).

20. *Nutr. Rev.,* **37,** 344 (1979).

21. J. L. B. Roepke and A. Kirskey, *Fed. Proc.,* **40,** 863 (1981).

22. P. E. Frye and L. E. Arnold, *Biol. Psychiat.,* **16,** 583 (1981).

2

Effects of Drugs on Cellular Transport of Nutrients

RICHARD F. BRANDA, M.D.

Department of Medicine, University of Minnesota, Minneapolis, Minnesota

Numerous clinically useful drugs have a profound effect on nutritional status by either enhancing or restricting the availability of nutrients. As these drug-nutrient interactions are studied in detail, it has become apparent that the mechanisms of drug action are highly diverse and often complex. Moreover, some drugs interact with nutrient metabolism in more than one way.

These complicated but important interactions of drugs and nutrients are well illustrated by the effects of drugs on folic acid metabolism. Investigation of these interactions has been intense for several reasons. First, folate deficiency causes serious hematologic disease. Folate compounds participate in nucleic acid, protein, and amino acid synthesis. Hence all dividing cells require folate coenzymes, and a deficiency of this vitamin due to dietary insufficiency or drug effect particularly impairs the rapidly proliferating cells of the bone marrow. Second, the folate analog methotrexate is widely used as a chemotherapeutic agent. Since methotrexate and physiologic folate compounds are usually handled similarly by the body, drugs that affect the metabolism of one compound are likely also to alter that of the other. Finally, a better understanding of drug-folate interactions provides basic insights into normal folate metabolism, particularly at the cellular level, and into how this metabolism can go awry in disease.

Attention was first drawn to the effects of drugs on folate metabolism when physicians noted anemia and other manifestations of folic acid de-

Work for this project was supported by a grant from the National Institutes of Health (CA 28234). Dr. Branda is the recipient of a Research Career Development Award (CA 00657).

13

ficiency in some patients receiving drugs. Further investigation showed that these drugs caused vitamin deficiency by different mechanisms (1). Thus drugs such as sulfasalazine interfere with intestinal absorption of the vitamin (2), whereas others (e.g., diphenylhydantoin) increase catabolism of folate compounds, and a third group, illustrated by the dihydrofolate reductase inhibitors trimethoprim and triamterene, block intracellular metabolism of folates (1).

More recently, interest has focused on the effects of drugs on the cellular transport of folate compounds. Since these studies for the most part have been performed in vitro with a variety of normal and neoplastic cell types, their results are not yet directly applicable at the bedside or the clinic. Nevertheless, they do provide fundamental information about the processes cells utilize to transport and incorporate folate compounds and they elucidate how these processes are altered by drugs. Eventually, this line of investigation should permit generalizations about drug structure–activity relationships which then can be used to predict the effects of drugs on cellular transport. The corollary of this proposition is that drugs might also be rationally selected or synthesized to manipulate this important cellular function.

CHARACTERISTICS OF MEMBRANE FOLATE TRANSPORT SYSTEMS

The membrane transport of folate compounds has been studied in a wide variety of normal and neoplastic cell types, ranging from bacterial to human origin (Table 1). Not surprisingly, the characteristics of folate transport differ importantly among the different cell types. Therefore,

Table 1. Some Cell Types Used to Study Transport and Metabolism of Folate Compounds in vitro

Normal	Neoplastic
Lactobacillus casei	Mouse L 1210 leukemia
Mouse intestinal epithelium	Murine leukemia cells (L 5178Y)
Rat hepatocytes	Murine Lewis lung tumor
Rat kidney	Ehrlich ascites tumor cells
Rabbit and hog choroid plexus	Sarcoma 180 cells
Rabbit reticulocytes	Human acute leukemia blasts
Human lymphoblastoid cell lines	Human breast cancer cells
Human lymphocytes	
Human bone marrow cells	
Human erythrocytes	

extrapolation of results obtained in one of these experimental systems to the situation in humans must be done cautiously. Additionally, interpretation of drug effects must be considered in the context of the cell type studied. For that reason, the characteristics of some of these systems are briefly outlined below. More extensive reviews are available (3–6).

Substrate Specificity

The ability of different folate transport systems to identify and selectively transfer folate compounds is highly variable. For example, *L. casei* appears to have a single transport system for all folate compounds, but excludes fragments of the folate molecule (4). Similarly, the oxidized folate compound pteroylglutamic acid or folic acid (PteGlu) can compete for transport with the physiologic, reduced forms of the vitamin in rabbit and hog choroid plexus (7, 8) and rat and hamster small intestine (2, 9–11), suggesting a shared transport system for oxidized and reduced folate compounds in these mammalian cell types. Like the *L. casei* system, neither pteroic acid nor tetrahydrobiopterin is transported by intestinal cells (2). In contrast, there appear to be two separate transport systems—one shared by reduced folate compounds and methotrexate, and a second for PteGlu—in murine L 1210 leukemia cells, Ehrlich ascites tumor cells, rabbit reticulocytes, cultured human breast cancer cells, phytohemagglutinin-stimulated human lymphocytes, and human erythrocytes (4, 12–17). In these cell types PteGlu is a poor inhibitor of reduced folate compound transport. Finally, rat hepatocytes appear to have complex, and perhaps multiple, systems for uptake of folate compounds. One system resembles murine leukemia cells, in that reduced folate compound and methotrexate transport are poorly inhibited by PteGlu, while a second system apparently transports reduced folates independently of methotrexate (18, 19). Overall, then, the membrane folate transport system requires a pteridine ring, the para-aminobenzoyl group, and at least one glutamate. This structural specificity is even higher in some cell membranes which can discriminate between oxidized and reduced folates, and between the very similar structures of PteGlu and methotrexate.

Saturability

In most cell types, transport of folate compounds is saturable (7–14, 16, 18). That is, incubation for cells with an increasing concentration of the compound results in increasing uptake but decreasing percentage incorporation, consistent with saturation of a membrane carrier system. A double reciprocal plot of uptake velocity against extracellular folate concentration results in a linear relationship typical of Michaelis-Menten kinetics. From such a plot, an affinity constant, K_m, and maximum transport velocity, V_{max}, can be determined. In some cell systems (rat intestine and hepatocytes, normal and leukemic human leukocytes), the uptake process is more complex; influx is saturable at low, but not at high, substrate concentrations (9, 18, 20). This second component of the uptake process may represent either a second, low-affinity transport system or simple passive diffusion of folate compounds at higher concentrations (18).

Affinity constants for 5-methyltetrahydrofolic acid are generally in the range of 1 μM, while slightly higher values are reported for other reduced folate compounds and methotrexate (4). In cell systems where reduced and oxidized forms of the vitamin appear to be transported separately (e.g., L 1210 leukemia cells), the transport constant for PteGlu is approximately 200 times higher (4). This indicates a much lower affinity carrier for this oxidized form of folate.

Temperature Dependence

In all cell types where it has been studied, folate compound transport is temperature sensitive, with Q_{10} values reported in the range of 2–8 (5, 13, 14, 21), except when very high external concentrations are used (20).

Energy Requirement

It is generally agreed that folate uptake is energy dependent and thus an active transport process. However, the effects of energy deprivation on transport differ markedly among the diverse cell types. For example, folate transport in L. casei is reduced by glucose restriction or metabolic inhibitors (4). Similarly, influx of folate compounds is decreased by metabolic inhibitors in rabbit choroid plexus, rat small intestine, and isolated hepatocytes (8, 10, 18). In contrast, metabolic poisons such as azide, iodoacetate, and 2,4-dinitrophenol actually increase steady-state levels of folate compounds in Sarcoma 180 cells, L 1210 leukemia cells, Ehrlich ascites tumor cells, rabbit reticulocytes, human acute myelogenous leukemia and breast cancer cells, and human erythrocytes (12–14, 16, 22, 23). This effect is reversed by exogenous glucose. Detailed studies suggest that this phenomenon is explained by inhibition of an energy-dependent efflux mechanism, which causes a net accumulation of folate compounds (23–25). However, the human erythrocyte may be an exception, since efflux rate is unchanged by nearly total depletion of ATP (16).

Concentrative Accumulation

Rat hepatocytes, L 1210 cells, rabbit choroid plexus, and human erythrocytes (8, 17, 18, 24) but not granulocytes (20) are able to concentrate folate compounds against an electrochemical gradient. In the case of L 1210 cells, this concentrative ability is greatly enhanced by the metabolic inhibitor azide presumably by its inhibiting the energy-dependent efflux mechanism described above (24).

Influence of Ionic Composition

Changes in the ionic composition of the suspending media can have either significant or no effect on folate transport, depending upon the cell type studied. Thus, transport is sodium dependent, and is inhibited by oubain in rat and hamster small intestine and in rat isolated hepatocytes (10, 11, 18, 19). Conversely, changes in sodium content of the media do not alter folate transport rates in hog choroid plexus, rabbit reticulocytes, or Ehrlich ascites tumor cells (7, 12, 14). Interestingly, the last-named cell types, plus human erythrocytes, exhibit increased folate transport when suspended in nonionic solutes such as sucrose or urea, suggesting that anions are inhibitory (12, 14, 26). This possibility has been explored in more detail, and it has been observed that a wide variety of inorganic and organic anions inhibit influx and net transport of folate compounds (12, 27).

Effects of pH

As might be predicted from the influence of ionic composition on folate transport described above, most anionic buffers alter membrane permeation of the vitamin, thereby necessitating the use of zwitterionic buffers for investigations of pH effect (28). Since this fact was only recently appreciated, it may account for the apparently conflicting effects of pH on folate transport. For example, low pH enhanced uptake of folate compounds by rat jejunum and Sarcoma 180 cells, but decreased transport by human leukocytes and bone marrow. In contrast, a broad pH optimum between 4.5 and 7.5 was observed for *L. casei* (11, 23, 29–31).

Our own studies with the human erythrocyte suggest that the direction of a pH gradient across the membrane is an important factor influencing the direction of net folate flux. Initial rates of uptake were inversely proportional to external pH. This effect was mediated by an enhancement of the affinity for folate compounds of the carrier (i.e., K_m decreased with lowering of the pH). In contrast, efflux increased with increasing external pH. Consequently, lowering the pH of the suspending medium markedly increased steady-state levels of 5-methyltetrahydrofolic acid (32).

INTERACTIONS OF DRUGS WITH THE FOLATE TRANSPORT SYSTEM

The evidence summarized above supports the concept that folate compounds are translocated across the cell membrane by a substrate-specific, carrier-mediated process. By analogy with other transport systems, this carrier most likely is a transmembrane protein embedded in membrane lipid, and preliminary characterization of this protein has been reported (4, 33–36). Because the transport process is complicated, there are multiple potential sites for interaction with drugs. For purposes of discussion, these drug effects will be arbitrarily divided into seven categories; however, these ascribed drug actions should be considered tentative and to some extent speculative. Additionally, some drugs almost certainly interact in more than one way.

Direct Competition for the Carrier

The folate transport system has high substrate specificity, and generally its affinity is highest for physiologic forms of the vitamin. Nevertheless, folate analogs are transported to a greater or lesser degree, and close analogs, such as methotrexate, are highly inhibitory (K_i of 7.7 μM in L 1210 cells) by directly competing for transport (4). Even drugs with more dissimilar structures, such as the dihydrofolate reductase inhibitor trimethoprim, can compete with 5-methyltetrahydrofolic acid for cellular uptake, but the degree of inhibition at clinically useful concentrations of trimethoprim is relatively weak (37).

Chemical Modification of the Transport Protein

Agents that react with sulfhydryl groups decrease the transport of reduced, but not oxidized, folate compounds in L 1210 leukemia cells, rat hepatocytes, human acute leukemia cells, and human erythrocytes (4, 17, 19, 22). This effect was seen with reagents which remain predominantly at the outside of the membrane as well as with those which react with both membrane and intracellular sulfhydryl groups (17). This finding has been interpreted to indicate that sulfhydryl groups, and perhaps intact disulfide bonds (18), are necessary for transport of folate compounds. In addition, the dichotomous effect of sulfhydryl reagents on the permeation of reduced and oxidized folate compounds is taken as further evidence that the membrane of these cells contains two separate mechanisms for their transport (3). Although the sulfhydryl reagents used in these studies are too toxic for clinical use, many commonly used drugs interact with sulfhydryl groups. Interestingly, one such agent, ethacrynic acid, was recently found by us to be a potent inhibitor of 5-methyltetrahydrofolic acid transport by red cells (38).

In addition to sulfhydryl groups, amino groups also appear to be important ligands at the transport site, at least in human erythrocytes. In this system, compounds that react with amino groups, such as pyridoxal phosphate and 4-acetamido-4'-isothiocyano-stilbene-2,2'-disulfonic acid (SITS), markedly inhibit transport of reduced, but not oxidized, folate compounds (17).

Inhibition by Anionic Compounds

Inorganic anions, organic anions, and anionic drugs (for example, acetylsalicylic acid, hydrocortisone, and cephalothin) inhibit uptake of folate compounds in nucleated cells (12, 22). The mechanism of this inhibition is unclear at present, and more than one mechanism may be operative. To better characterize these drug effects, we used the human erythrocyte as a model system, since its membrane is relatively simple and well characterized.

We first considered the most direct explanation of this inhibition: that anions compete with folate compounds at a common transport site. In the red cell, anion transport is associated with the transmembrane protein, band 3 (39), and the characteristics of both inorganic (chloride, sulfate, phosphate) and organic (lactate) anion transfer have been well defined (40, 41). A comparison of these three permeation systems is

Table 2. Comparison of Anion Transport Pathways of the Erythrocyte

	5-Methyltetra-hydrofolic acid	Inorganic Anions[a] $(PO_4^{2-}, SO_4^{2-}$	Organic Anions (Lactate)
pH	Inverse relationship	Max at pH 6.5	Inverse relationship
Species sequence	Guinea pig, sheep, man, rabbit, pig	Sheep, pig, man, guinea pig, rabbit	
Chemical modifications	— (% Inhibition) —		
pCMBS (10^{-4} M)	40	0	65
Pronase (2.5 mg/ml)	10	0	47
Carbodiimide (25 mM)	30	52	35
Bimodal inhibitors	— Concentration (mM) for 50% Inhibition of Transfer —		
Pyridoxal phosphate	0.3	1	5
SITS	0.15	0.02	0.20
DIDS	>0.01	0.001	—
Reversible inhibitors			
Dipyridamole	0.025	0.006	—
Ethacrynic acid	0.04	0.5	—
Phlorizin	1.0	0.55	<0.6
Procaine	6	0.3	—
Chlopromazine	>0.5	0.25	<0.6

[a]Modified from data published by Deuticke and co-workers (40,41).

summarized in Table 2. These investigations led us to conclude that while there are remarkable similarities between these carriers, the erythrocyte has separate transport systems for anions and folate compounds, since: (1) the species sequences for anion and folate transport are entirely different (42); (2) guinea pig erythrocytes are freely permeable to anions but nearly impermeable to folate compounds (40, 42); (3) proteolytic enzymes decrease anion but not folate transport (17); and (4) the highly specific and potent inhibitor of anion transport, 4,4'-diisothiocyano-2,2'-stilbene disulfonate (DIDS), is only a weak inhibitor of folate transport (17).

Although it thus appears that anions and folate compounds do not share a permeation pathway, further observations, in addition to the inhibitory activity of anions, indicate that the two carriers are structurally or functionally related. For example, agents known to interact with band 3 and to inhibit anion transport (43, 44) also decrease uptake of 5-methyltetrahydrofolic acid. Dipyridamole, pyridoxal phosphate, SITS, and phlorizin decrease incorporation of the vitamin by 60–80%

Table 3.   Amphipathic Drugs Inhibit 5-Methyltetrahydrofolic Acid Uptake by Human Red Cells

Drug	Concentration (mM) for 50 % Inhibition of Uptake[a]	Uptake Inhibition (%) at Pharmacologically Relevant Concentrations	pKa
Dipryidamole	0.025	22.7 (9.6–43.4)[b]	6.3
Ethacrynic acid	0.040	12.8 (0–18.4	3.5
Sulfinpyrazone	0.100	31.3 (28.8–34.4)	2.8
Phenylbutazone	0.750	43.8 (39.2–48.4)	4.5
Furosemide	0.800	9.4 (0–19)	3.9
Phlorizin	1.0	—	7.3
Sodium barbitol			
	2.5	7.4 (4–12.2)	8.5
Procaine	5.5	0	8.7
Chlopromazine	>0.5	0	9.3

[a]Data from Branda and Nelson (38).
[b]Mean (range).

(17). Furthermore, drugs previously found to inhibit anion transport also decrease folate uptake (38). As shown in Table 3, all drugs in this category which were tested were to some extent inhibitory, but only anionic amphipathic (that is, molecules with anionic-apolar character) were highly active at pharmacologically relevant concentrations. Consequently, inhibitory activity correlated with drug dissociation constant ($r = 0.87$). A double-reciprocal plot analysis of drug effect on 5-methyltetrahydrofolic acid transport showed changes in both K_m and V_{max} (indicating a mixture of competitive and noncompetitive inhibition) by ethacrynic acid, sulfasalazine, and phlorizin (38).

To analyze in more detail the relationship between the physicochemical and inhibitory properties of these drugs, we also measured the inhibitory activity of a series of eight phenoxyacetic derivatives, including ethacrynic acid (Table 4). The inhibitory activities of the compounds are expressed as log I_{50} (log of the molar concentration producing 50% inhibition, computed graphically by plotting molar concentration versus mean uptake inhibition). This inhibitory activity strongly correlates ($r = 0.87$) with the liposolubility of the drug (38) as quantified by the $R_M H_2 O$ (45). The electronic effects of substituents also have some influence on activity, since inhibition and σ are correlated ($r = 0.56$) (38). Thus, groups that attract electrons also increase inhibitory activity.

Table 4. Physiochemical Properties and Inhibitory Activities of Phenoxyacetic Acid Derivatives on 5-CH₃-H₄-Folic Acid Transport

Compounds	Formula	$\log I_{50}$*	R_{MH_2O}[δ']	σ[δ"]
Ethacrynic Acid	C_2H_5 CH_2 CCO Cl Cl OCH_2COOH	4.40	2.09	1.03
4 Chlorophenoxyacetic Acid	Cl OCH_2COOH	2.89	0.99	0.23
2,3 Dichlorophenoxyacetic Acid	Cl Cl OCH_2COOH	2.52	1.36	0.60
2,4 Dichlorophenoxyacetic Acid	Cl, Cl OCH_2COOH	2.22	1.39	0.46
2 Nitrophenoxyacetic Acid	NO_2 OCH_2COOH	2.02	0.40	0.78
3 Methylphenoxyacetic Acid	CH_3 OCH_2COOH	2.00	0.88	-0.07
P-acetylphenoxyacetic Acid	CH_3CO OCH_2COOH	1.19	0.45	0.50
Phenoxyacetic Acid	OCH_2COOH	1.60	0.37	0

* Values computed graphically, as described in the text, from the means of at least 3 separate experiments performed in triplicate.

δ From Motais and Cousin (45).

' A measure of partition data equivalent to the logarithm of the partition coefficient (see ref. 46).

" σ is defined by the equation: $\log K/K_o = \rho\sigma$, where K is a constant describing a reaction of substituted aromatic compound, K_o is the constant for the parent compound, and ρ is a constant characteristic of the reaction (45).

These observations indicate that predictions about the inhibitory activity of a drug can be made from its structural characteristics, and that most compounds that inhibit erythrocyte membrane anion transfer have qualitatively, but not necessarily quantitatively, similar effects on folate transport.

Our studies to date cannot exclude a structural relationship between anion and folate transport in the red cell membrane to account for the observed anion inhibitory and drug effects. For example, if band 3 represents a family of transport proteins, agents that interfere with band 3 function might affect both systems. There is no direct evidence to substantiate this association at present. In fact, we recently had the opportunity to study a patient with markedly reduced folate transport, and in this case the intramembrane particles, which are thought to be composed primarily of band 3 protein, were normal in size and distribution. In addition, band 3 migration in SDS polyacrylamide gel electrophoresis was normal (47). It is possible, however, that a more subtle structural abnormality of band 3 was present in this patient.

A third possibility, and the one one we currently favor, is that anion and folate transport are functionally coupled, probably to maintain electrochemical neutrality in the cell. In this case drugs or environmental changes that affect one transport system would indirectly affect the other. To study this putative functional relationship, we first confirmed in the mature erythrocyte that chloride inhibits folate compound permeation (14), since this seemed to be the simplest model of the interaction of anion and folate transport. We found that chloride ion competitively inhibits membrane transport of 5-methyltetrahydrofolic acid, and that establishment of an outwardly directed chloride gradient by incubation of erythrocytes in isotonic sucrose or by treatment with the chloride ionophore tributyltin increases folate permeation (26). Additional studies indicate that this effect of a chloride gradient is indeed indirect, produced by generation of a pH gradient. Creation of an outwardly directed chloride gradient lowers extracellular pH by exchanging for OH^- (48). We have previously shown that the direction of a pH gradient across the membrane is an important factor influencing the direction of net folate flux, and that the effects of pH on folate transport are consistent with coupled OH^- exchange or H^+ co-permeation (32). Consequently, our data support the notion that in the presence of a chloride gradient, H^+-folate co-permeation is driven by a pH gradient. In partial confirmation of this mechanism, we have recently found that the carbonic anhydrase inhibitor acetazolamide blocks the stimulatory effect of a chloride gradient on folate transport. Our preliminary conclusion, therefore, is that drugs which inhibit anion transport may simultaneously affect 5-methyltetrahydrofolic acid transport in the red cell by altering the functional interactions of these two permeation systems.

Using isolated brush border membranes from rat kidney, Selhub and co-workers described an entirely different mechanism for the inhibitory effects of anions. They found that anions such as chloride stabilize the association between 5-methyltetrahydrofolic acid and a membrane folate-binding protein, thereby decreasing the rate of exchange with exogenous folate (49).

Alteration of pH

Uptake of folate compounds by rat jejunum, Sarcoma 180 cells, and human erythrocytes is inhibited by elevating the pH of the suspending medium (11, 23, 32). Consequently, a drug that imparts an alkaline pH to its solution when dissolved might thereby impair folate transport. This mechanism has been invoked to explain the low serum folate levels that frequently occur in patients receiving diphenylhydantoin (2). However, whether this drug alkalinizes the intestinal lumen during clinical use is controversial; moreover, another mechanism of drug action (increased catabolism of folate) has also been described (1).

Changes of Membrane Lipids

In an interesting experiment, L 1210 cells were grown in host animals fed diets rich in either saturated or polyunsaturated fat (50). This dietary manipulation resulted in changes of the lipid composition of the leukemic cell membranes, with greater membrane fluidity in cells grown in animals fed the unsaturated fat diet. Measurements of methotrexate transport showed that permeability was considerably greater in cells with more fluid membranes; K_m was lowered, but V_{max} was unchanged. This study suggests that changes in membrane lipid structure and physical properties brought about by dietary modification can alter the transport of folate compounds.

A second approach used to modify membrane lipid composition is to introduce charged liposomes (51). Positively charged liposomes were found to increase bidirectional methotrexate fluxes in Ehrlich ascites tumor cells, but there was no effect on steady-state levels. Kinetic analysis showed that V_{max} was increased but K_m was unchanged. In contrast, negatively charged liposomes reduced methotrexate influx. Besides contributing to an understanding of the interaction between membrane transport carriers and their lipid environment, these studies are relevant to the increasing use of liposomes as drug carriers (52).

Inhibition of Folate Efflux

A characteristic of many folate transport systems is that metabolic inhibitors cause an increase of steady-state levels of the vitamin, presumably by inhibiting an energy-dependent efflux mechanism (23–25). While metabolic poisons such as azide, cyanide, and 2,4-dinitrophenol are obviously of no clinical use, some drugs have a similar effect on folate compound efflux. The vinca alkaloids vincristine and vinblastine increase net uptake of methotrexate in Ehrlich ascites tumor cells, L 1210 leukemia, and human acute myelogenous leukemia cells, but not in mouse fibroblasts or isolated intestinal epithelial cells (22, 53–55). This possible selectivity engendered a hope that the combination of vincristine and methotrexate would be synergistic against leukemic but not against normal cells. When this possibility was tested in vivo, only additive effects of the chemotherapeutic agents were found if vincristine was administered prior to or together with methotrexate (55, 56), but some synergism was seen if the vincristine was delayed 24 hours or more (55).

The organic acid probenecid also increases the steady-state level of intracellular methotrexate in L 1210 cells, Sarcoma 180 cells, and Ehrlich carcinoma cells (57). While this drug inhibits both influx and efflux, the concentration required to inhibit influx is ten times greater than that required to inhibit efflux. Consequently, at pharmacologically relevant concentrations, efflux is inhibited to a greater extent (57). This observation has been extended to show that the combination of probenecid plus methotrexate is more effective than the latter drug alone to increase life span of mice bearing L 1210 leukemia (58). Probenecid also prolongs the cerebrospinal fluid half-life of methotrexate in humans, again by inhibiting exit of the drug (59).

Alteration of Cyclic Nucleotide Levels

In 1973, Hoffbrand and co-workers found that high concentrations of dibutyryl cyclic AMP and phosphodiesterase inhibitors such as theophylline (which raises intracellular cyclic AMP) inhibited uptake of methotrexate into phytohaemagglutinin-stimulated lymphocytes (60). Similar effects of these drugs were seen on 50-methyltetrahydrofolic acid but not PteGlu uptake. Based on these findings, the authors proposed that cyclic AMP concentrations may have a controlling effect on methotrexate and reduced folate compound entry. Their studies were extended by Huennekens and associates in L 1210 cells. They found that several different phosphodiesterase inhibitors (1-methyl-3-isobutylxanthine, theophylline) and adenylate cyclase stimulators (histamine, prostaglandins E_1 and E_2) inhibited methotrexate uptake (4). Moreover, an inverse relationship between cyclic AMP levels and rates of methotrexate transport was noted. They also concluded that methotrexate transport is regulated by the intracellular level of cyclic AMP.

More recently, a third group has published studies in Ehrlich ascites tumor cells suggesting that the changes in methotrexate transport and cyclic AMP levels, when they occur together, may be coincidental (61). They found that levels of cyclic AMP could be increased by cholera toxin without altering methotrexate influx, and that changes in cell cyclic AMP levels and inhibition of methotrexate influx were temporally dissociated, In addition, they reported that changes in methotrexate transport could occur without significant changes in cyclic AMP levels. Consequently, the regulatory function of cyclic nucleotides on folate compound transport is uncertain at present.

CONCLUSION

Folate compound incorporation into cells is a useful model for studies of the effects of drugs on cellular transport of nutrients because the transport process has been well characterized. Permeation appears to be mediated by a protein carrier or channel embedded in membrane lipid. In most cell types, transport is substrate specific, saturable, temperature and energy dependent, concentrative, and influenced by the ionic composition and pH of the surrounding solution. However, both qualitative and quantitative differences in these characteristics can occur among cells of different tissue and species origins. Since the transport process is complicated, drugs can interact by multiple mechanisms. In this discussion, drug effects are divided into seven categories: (1) direct competition for the carrier; (2) chemical modification of the transport protein; (3) inhibition by anionic compounds; (4) alteration of pH; (5) changes of membrane lipids; (6) inhibition of folate efflux; and (7) modification of cyclic nucleotide levels. While examples of each type of drug effect are cited, it is likely that many, and perhaps most, drugs have more than one action. For example, ethacrynic acid is a potent inhibitor of 5-methyltetrahydrofolic acid transport by human erythrocytes. This inhibitory activity can be related to its reactivity with sulfhydryl groups, its lipid solubility, and its anionic nature at physiologic pH.

While these in vitro studies are valuable to define drug structure-activity relationships and further elucidate the folate transport mechanism, their results can not be extrapolated directly to the patient. Other factors, such as plasma protein binding, and complex interactions of drug and vitamin absorption, metabolism, and excretion will also influence drug effects in vivo. Nevertheless, it seems likely that drugs identified by these approaches may alter the metabolism and distribution of folate compounds in some patients.

REFERENCES

1. J. M. Scott and D. G. Weir, *Clinics Haematol.*, **9**, 587 (1980).
2. I. H. Rosenberg, *Clinics Haematol.*, **5**, 589 (1976).
3. F. M. Huennekens, P. M. DiGirolamo, K. Fujii, G. B. Henderson, D. W. Jacobsen, V. G. Neef, and J. I. Rader, *Adv. Enzyme Regul.*, **12**, 131 (1974).
4. F. M. Huennekens, K. S. Vitols, and G. B. Henderson, *Adv. Enzymology*, **47**, 313 (1978).
5. F. M. Sirotnak, *Pharmac. Ther.*, **8**, 71 (1980).
6. B. A. Kamen and J. R. Bertino, *Antibiotics Chemother.*, **28**, 62 (1980).
7. C. P. Chen and C. Wagner, *Life Sciences*, **16**, 1571 (1975).
8. R. Spector and A. V. Lorenzo, *Science*, **187**, 540 (1975).
9. J. Selhub and I. H. Rosenberg, *J. Biol. Chem.*, **256**, 4489 (1981).
10. R. C. Rose, M. J. Koch, and D. L. Nahrwold, *Am. J. Physiol.*, **235**, E678 (1979).
11. W. B. Strum, *Biochim. Biophys. Acta*, **554**, 249 (1979).
12. I. D. Goldman, *Ann. N.Y. Acad. Sci.*, **186**, 400 (1971).
13. R. L. Schilsky, B. D. Bailey, and B. A. Chabner, *Biochem. Pharm.*, **30**, 1537 (1981).
14. W. F. Bobzien and I. D. Goldman, *J. Clin. Invest.*, **51**, 1688 (1972).
15. K. C. Das and A. V. Hoffbrand, *Br. J. Haematol.*, **19**, 203 (1970).
16. R. F. Branda, B. K. Anthony, and H. S. Jacob, *J. Clin. Invest.*, **61**, 1270 (1978).
17. R. F. Branda and B. K. Anthony, *J. Lab. Clin. Med.*, **94**, 354 (1979).
18. D. W. Horne, W. T. Briggs, and C. Wagner, *J. Biol. Chem.*, **253**, 3529 (1978).
19. D. A. Gewirtz, J. C. White, J. K. Randolph, and I. D. Goldman, *Cancer Res.*, **40**, 573 (1980).
20. D. Kessel, T. C. Hall, and De. W. Roberts, *Cancer Res.*, **28**, 564 (1968)
21. A. Nahas, P. F. Nixon, and J. R. Bertino, *Cancer Res.*, **32**, 1416 (1972).
22. R. A. Bender, *Cancer Chemo. Reports*, Part 3, Vol. 6, 73 (1975).
23. M. T. Hakala, *Biochim. Biophys. Acta*, **102**, 210 (1965).
24. I. D. Goldman, *J. Biol. Chem.*, **244**, 3779 (1969).
25. D. W. Fry, J. C. White, and I. D. Goldman, *Cancer Res.*, **40**, 3669 (1980).
26. R. F. Branda and N. L. Nelson, *Proceedings XII Inter. Congress of Nutrition*, in press.
27. J. C. Jennette and I. D. Goldman, *J. Lab. Clin. Med.*, **86**, 834 (1975).
28. G. B. Henderson and E. M. Zevely, *Arch. Biochem. Biophys.*, **200**, 149 (1980).
29. D. Kessel and T. C. Hall, *Biochem. Pharm.*, **16**, 2395 (1967).
30. J. J. Corcino, S. Waxman, and V. Herbert, *Br. J. Haematol.*, **20**, 503 (1971).
31. G. B. Henderson and F. M. Huennekens, *Arch. Biochem. Biophys.*, **164**, 722 (1974).
32. R. F. Branda and N. L. Nelson, Submitted for publication.
33. G. B. Henderson, E. M. Zevely, and F. M. Huennekens, *J. Biol. Chem.*, **252**, 3760 (1977).
34. R. Spector, *J. Biol. Chem.*, **252**, 3364 (1977).
35. M. M. Zamierowski and C. Wagner, *J. Biol. Chem.*, **252**, 933 (1977).
36. A. C. Antony, C. Utley, K. C. VanHorne, and J. F. Kolhouse, *J. Biol. Chem.*, **256**, 9684 (1981).
37. D. Neithammer and R. C. Jackson, *Br. J. Haematol.*, **32**, 273 (1976).

38. R. F. Branda and N. L. Nelson, *Drug-Nutrient Interactions*, **1**, 45 (1981).

39. Z. I. Cabantchik and A. Rothstein, *J. Membr. Biol.*, **15**, 207 (1974).

40. B. Deuticke, *Rev. Physiol. Biochem. Pharmacol.*, **78**, 1 (1977).

41. B. Deuticke, I. Rickert, and E. Beyer, *Biochim. Biophys. Acta*, **507**, 137 (1978).

42. R. F. Branda, *J. Nutrition*, **111**, 618 (1981).

43. A. Rothstein and P. A. Knauf, *Adv. Exp. Med. Biol.*, **84**, 319 (1977).

44. S. Lepke and H. Passow, *Biochim. Biophys. Acta*, **298**, 529 (1973).

45. R. Motais and J. L. Cousin, in R. W. Straub and L. Bolis, Eds., *Cell Membrane Receptors for Drugs and Hormones: A Multidisciplinary Approach*, Raven, New York, 1978, p. 219.

46. R. Motais and J. L. Cousin, *Am. J. Physiol.*, **231**, 1485 (1976).

47. R. B. Howe, R. F. Branda, S. D. Douglas, and R. D. Brunning, *Blood*, **54**, 1080 (1979).

48. E. J. Fitzsimons and J. Sendroy, *J. Biol. Chem.*, **236**, 1595 (1961).

49. J. Selhub, A. C. Gay, and I. H. Rosenberg, *Biochim. Biophys. Acta*, **557**, 372 (1979).

50. C. P. Burns, D. G. Luttenegger, D. T. Dudley, G. R. Buettner, and A. A. Spector, *Cancer Res.*, **39**, 1926 (1979).

51. D. W. Fry, J. C. White, and I. D. Goldman, *J. Membrane Biol.*, **50**, 123 (1979).

52. J. N. Weinstein, R. L. Magin, M. B. Yatvin, and D. S. Zaharko, *Science*, **204**, 188 (1979).

53. R. F. Zager, S. A. Frisby, and V. T. Oliverio, *Cancer Res.*, **33**, 1670 (1973).

54. M. J. Fyfe, and I. D. Goldman, *J. Biol. Chem.*, **248**, 5067 (1973).

55. P. L. Chello, F. M. Sirotnak, and D. M. Dorick, *Cancer Res.*, **39**, 2106 (1979).

56. R. A. Bender, A. P. Nichols, L. Norton, and R. M. Simon, *Cancer Treat. Reports*, **62**, 997 (1978).

57. F. M. Sirotnak, D. M. Moccio, and C. W. Young, *Cancer Res.*, **41**, 966 (1981).

58. F. M. Sirotnak, D. M. Moccio, C. H. Hancock, and C. W. Young, *Cancer Res.*, **41**, 3944 (1981).

59. U. Bode, I. T. Magrath, W. A. Bleyer, D. G. Poplack, and D. L. Glaubiger, *Cancer Res.*, **40**, 2184 (1980).

60. A. V. Hoffbrand, E. Tripp, D. Catovsky, and K. C. Das, *Br. J. Haematol.*, **25**, 497 (1973).

61. J. C. White, R. A. Carchman, D. W. Fry, and I. D. Goldman, *Cancer Res.*, **40**, 2400 (1980).

3

Vitamin D Metabolism and Metabolic Bone Disease

ZANE N. GAUT, M.D., Ph.D.

Hoffman-La Roche, Inc., Nutley, New Jersey

The discovery that vitamin D (Figure 1) is not itself active but must be metabolically activated before it can function led to the discovery that the kidney is the site of production of a very potent hormone derived from the vitamin (1–4). Further elucidation of this discovery described the vitamin D endocrine system based in the kidney (Figure 2). In this system, it is now apparent that the need for calcium and phosphorus stimulates either the production or the accumulation of 1,25-dihydroxyvitamin D_3 [1,25-$(OH)_2D_3$]. The 1,25-$(OH)_2D_3$ then stimulates the absorption of calcium and phosphorus from the intestinal contents and, perhaps in concert with parathyroid hormone, mobilizes calcium and phosphorus from bone. These discoveries provided a new understanding of such diseases as renal osteodystrophy, various types of hypoparathyroidism, and certain types of vitamin D-resistant rickets. They also provided new insights into the development of postmenopausal osteoporosis which was recently reviewed by DeLuca and co-workers (5).

Since the usefulness of calcitriol in the treatment of renal osteodystrophy and various types of hypoarathryoidism is well established, this chapter will focus primarily on the metabolism of vitamin D, the potential usefulness of calcitriol in the treatment of postmenopausal osteoporosis, and the pharmacokinetics of calcitriol.

Appreciation is expressed to Ms. Ruth Wyler, Ms. Betty Holland, Ms. Marilyn Kozak, and Dr. Milan Uskokovic for technical advice and valuable assistance.

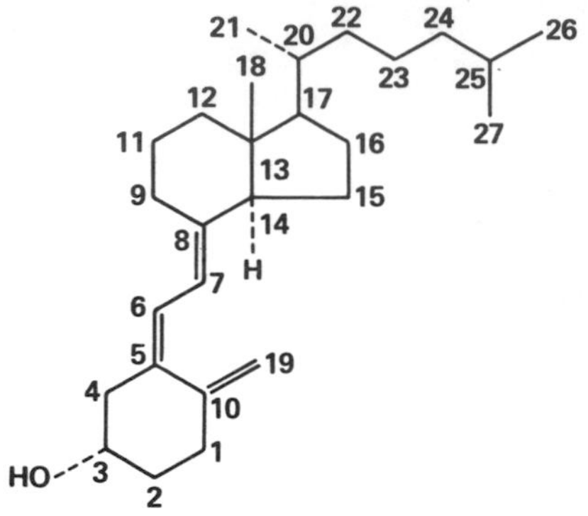

Figure 1. Structure of vitamin D_3 and its carbon numbering system.

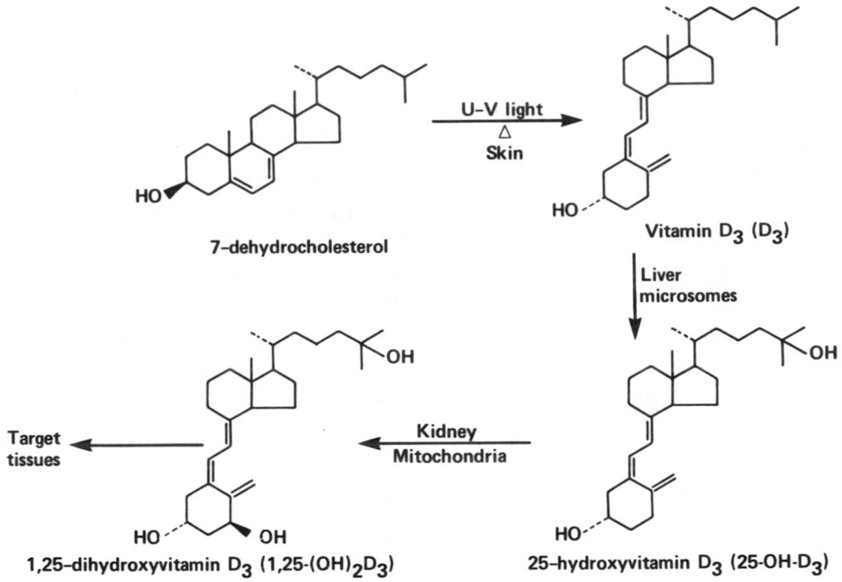

7-dehydrocholesterol

U-V light
Δ
Skin

Vitamin D_3 (D_3)

Liver microsomes

1,25-dihydroxyvitamin D_3 (1,25-(OH)$_2$D$_3$)

Target tissues

Kidney Mitochondria

25-hydroxyvitamin D_3 (25-OH-D$_3$)

Reference: H. F. DeLuca, Curr. Med. Res. Opin. 7 (5): 279-293, 1981.

Figure 2. Production and metabolism of vitamin D_3 necessary for its biological activity.

THE VITAMIN D ENDOCRINE SYSTEM

Many of the structures of the metabolically active forms of vitamin D have been defined, as have the organs involved in their conversions. Vitamin D is produced in the epidermis by ultraviolet irradiation of 7-dehydrocholesterol (Figure 2). This purely photolytic reaction produces previtamin D, which slowly isomerizes to vitamin D_3. Vitamin D_3 is then bound to the plasma transport protein and is transferred to the liver for further activation (6, 7). Alternatively, vitamin D_3 can be absorbed in the distal small intestine and transferred primarily through the lacteal system to be cleared by the liver. In the endoplasmic reticulum of the liver, vitamin D_3 is converted to 25-hydroxyvitamin D_3 (25-OH-D_3) by a mixed-function mono-oxygenase that is dependent upon a cytochrome P-450 (8–10). This cytochrome P-450, however, is not induced by phenobarbital and phenytoin. In addition to the microsomal 25-hydroxylase, a mitochondrial 25-hydroxylase also exists (11, 12). This enzyme has a much higher Michaelis constant for vitamin D_3 and is not specific for vitamin D_3 since it also hydroxylates cholesterol. It is likely, therefore, that under conditions where large amounts of vitamin D are administered, the mitochondrial 25-hydroxylase also operates, eliminating the impact of product suppression of the microsomal 25-hydroxylase (13). The intestine and kidney can also produce 25-OH-D_3, although the amounts of 25-hydroxylation taking place in these organs is small (14, 15). In addition, hepatectomized animals administered radioactive vitamin D_3 convert only small amounts to 25-OH-D_3 (16,17). Thus, the liver can be considered the major site of 25-hydroxylation of vitamin D_3 under physiological conditions.

The 25-OH-D_3 is then transported to the kidney on the vitamin D transport globulin where it can be converted to a variety of compounds, of which the most important appears to be 1,25-$(OH)_2D_3$. This reaction occurs in the mitochondrial fraction and is catalyzed by a three-component, mixed-function mono-oxygenase involving NADPH, molecular oxygen, a flavoprotein, an iron-sulfur protein, and a cytochrome P-450 (18–20). Like the 25-hydroxylase, this cytochrome P-450 is not induced by phenobarbital and phenytoin. The cytochrome P-450 portion of this hydroxylase is regulated by the need for calcium, phosphorus, and other regulatory factors. The 1,25-$(OH)_2D_3$ is then transported to the intestine, bone, and kidney, where it carries out its functions. In vivo, the mobilization of calcium from bone and possibly the renal reabsorption of calcium require the presence of parathyroid hormone, whereas the function in the intestine does not require the peptide hormone once 1,25-$(OH)_2D_3$ is formed (21).

The key experiment that demonstrates the essential role of the kidney for vitamin D function is that anephric rats or man do not respond in terms of intestinal calcium transport or bone calcium mobilization to a physiological dose of 25-OH-D_3 whereas they fully respond to 1,25-$(OH)_2D_3$. These experiments clearly demonstrate that 1,25-$(OH)_2D_3$ or a further metabolite, and not its precursor,

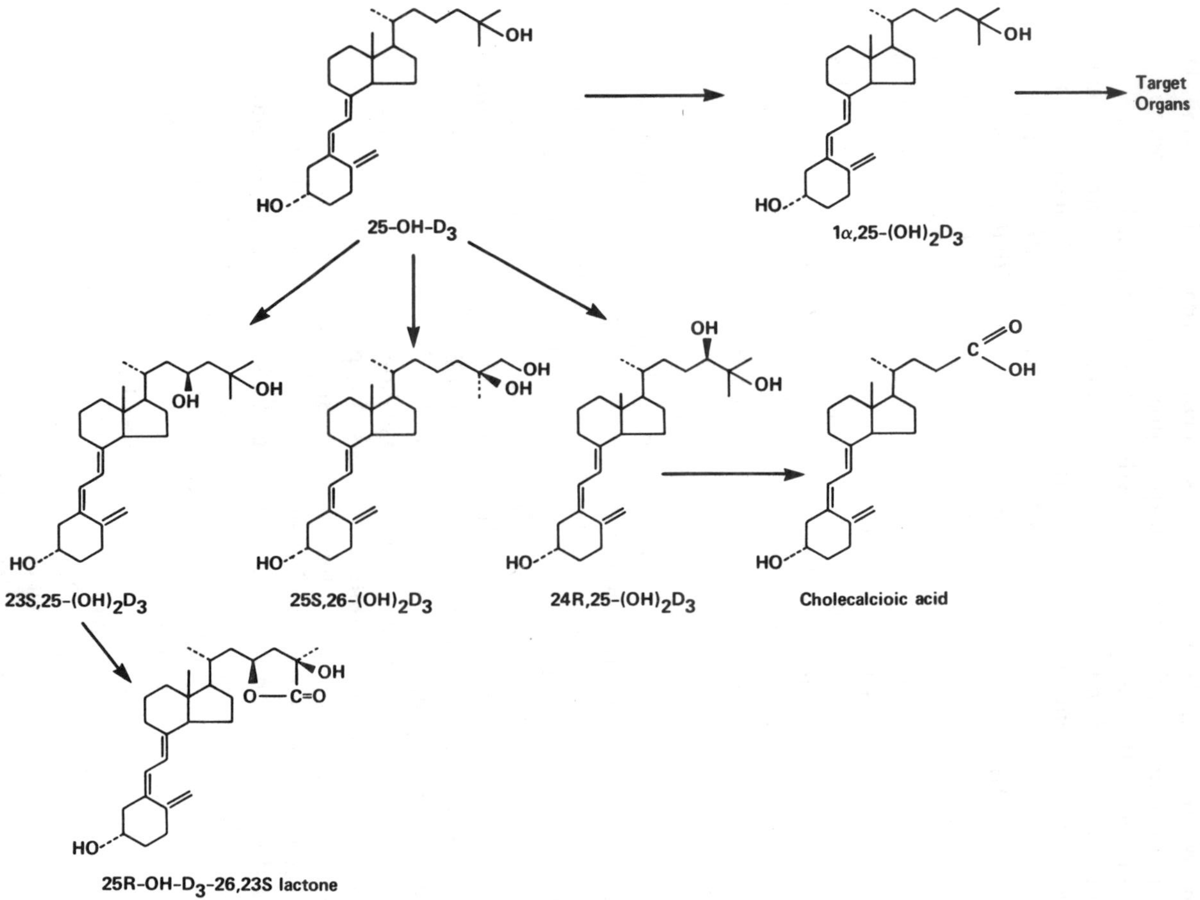

Figure 3. Metabolism of 25-OH-D₃ by the kidney.

25-OH-D_3, is the physiologically active form of the vitamin in these systems (22, 23).

The possibility remains, however, that vitamin D has other functions that may involve either other metabolites or a heretofore unknown function of 1,25-$(OH)_2D_3$. An example of that possibility is the 24R-hydroxylation of 25-OH-D_3 (Figure 3). This reaction occurs in the kidney, intestine, and cartilage tissue to produce the compound 24R,25-dihydroxyvitamin D_3 [24R,25-$(OH)_2D_3$] (24–26). It has been suggested that this compound is responsible for the mineralization of bone (27, 28), for the suppression of parathyroid hormone secretion, for the production of cartilaginous components (29), and for the development of chick embryos (30). So far, these functions have not been proved and, in fact, considerable evidence is now accumulating against the so-called mineralization requirement for 24R,25-$(OH)_2D_3$. With the use of 24,24-difluoro-25-hydroxyvitamin D_3 (24,24-F_2-25-OH-D_3) (Figure 4), a compound that cannot be 24-hydroxylated, it has been possible to demonstrate that 24R-hydroxylation is not required for 25-OH-D_3 to effect normal mineralization (31–34). In fact, the most potent mineralizing analog of vitamin D known is 24,24-difluoro-1,25-dihydroxyvitamin D_3 (24,24-F_2-1,25-$(OH)_2D_3$) (31). The kidney also converts 25-OH-D_3 to three other known compounds (Figure 2). They are 25-OH-D_3-26,23-lactone (35,36), 25S,26-dihydroxyvitamin D_3 (37), and 23,25-dihydroxyvitamin D_3 (Tanaka and DeLuca, unpublished results) (Figure 3).

The role of these compounds in the function or inactivation of vitamin D has not yet been fully evaluated. However, these compounds have weak biological activity in the known systems responsive to vitamin D. Thus, if they have significant physiological roles, these remain to be discovered. For the purpose of this discussion, therefore, attention will be focused on the 1,25-$(OH)_2D_3$ system.

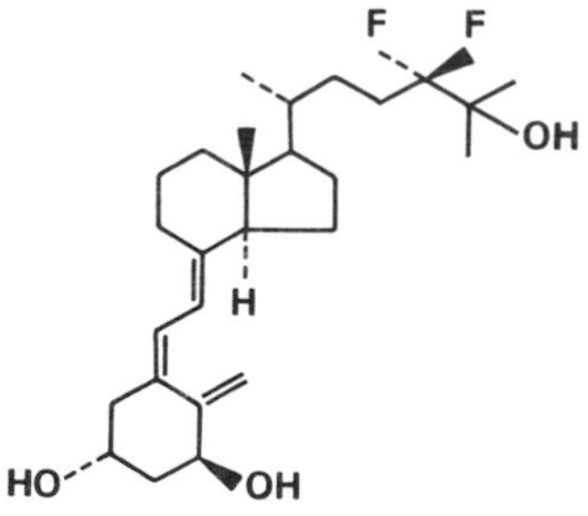

Figure 4.   Structure of 1-alpha-25$(OH)_2$-24,24$(F)_2$-D_3 (Ro 22-9343).

In true hormonal fashion, the production of $1,25\text{-(OH)}_2D_3$ is regulated by the need for calcium (38). Thus, hypocalcemic animals and man under otherwise normal conditions manifest high concentrations of $1,25\text{-(OH)}_2D_3$ in the plasma. Animals on a low-calcium diet upon parathyroidectomy lose the ability to increase their plasma levels of $1,25\text{-(OH)}_2D_3$ in response to the need for calcium (39). Injection of parathyroid hormone into parathyroidectomized rats will markedly stimulate 1-hydroxylation and suppress 24-hydroxylation of 25-OH-D_3 (39,40). In support of this, hyperparathyroid patients show high levels of $1,25\text{-(OH)}_2D_3$, whereas hypoparathyroid patients show low levels (8). Thus, the vitamin D system appears to have the parathyroid gland as an important regulator. In response to calcium deprivation, the secreted parathyroid hormone stimulates the $25\text{-OH-D}_3\text{-}1\text{-alpha-hydroxylase}$ in the kidney. The $1,25\text{-(OH)}_2D_3$ thus produced stimulates intestinal calcium absorption and, in concert with parathyroid hormone, stimulates the mobilization of calcium from bone (21). Likewise, the two hormones function in concert in stimulating renal conservation of calcium in the distal tubule (41, 42). These systems then bring about elevation of the plasma calcium to normal levels that then suppress parathyroid hormone secretion.

In addition to the parathyroid hormone complex, the production of $1,25\text{-(OH)}_2D_3$ is stimulated by hypophosphatemia (43), and is suppressed by $1,25\text{-(OH)}_2D_3$ itself (44). The 1-alpha-hydroxylase is also stimulated either directly or indirectly by growth hormone (45), possibly by prolactin (46), and in some species by the sex hormones estrogen, testosterone, and progesterone (36,46,47). The cellular and molecular mechanisms whereby the $25\text{-OH-D}_3\text{-}1\text{-alpha-hydroxylase}$ is regulated remain unknown, despite the development of in vitro primary cultures of kidney cells that carry out these conversions and illustrate some of the regulatory phenomena (48,49). For the purpose of this discussion, however, it is essential to remember that parathyroid hormone represents the major stimulator of $1,25\text{-(OH)}_2D_3$ production, phosphate may be a suppressant of $1,25\text{-(OH)}_2D_3$ production, and certain hormones, such as growth hormone, estrogen, and possibly prolactin, could function to facilitate the renal production of $1,25\text{-(OH)}_2D_3$. A final point to remember is that the placenta also possesses the $25\text{-OH-D}_3\text{-}1\text{-alpha-hydroxylase}$ (50).

POSTMENOPAUSAL OSTEOPOROSIS

This disease is quite complex (51,52) and, in all probability, does not rest on any single biochemical basis. However, there are two interesting facts to keep in mind. There is an age-related decrease in intestinal calcium absorption that correlates with plasma levels of $1,25\text{-}(OH)_2D_3$ (53,54). Aged patients and animals will respond to exogenous doses of $1,25\text{-}(OH)_2D_3$ in terms of elevation of intestinal calcium absorption. Thus, in aged patients, there is capacity for intestinal calcium absorption that can be stimulated by $1,25\text{-}(OH)_2D_3$. A second fact is that postmenopausal females suffering from osteoporosis have lower rates of calcium absorption than their age- and sex-matched controls (55). Analysis of plasma levels of $1,25\text{-}(OH)_2D_3$ has revealed that these values are approximately 30% lower than in age- and sex-matched controls, correlating with their failure of intestinal calcium absorption. Increased calcium absorption in response to the need for calcium is an essential physiological protective mechanism for the skeleton (32,56). This regulatory phenomenon may very well be significant in the appearance of postmenopausal osteoporosis (32,53–56).

Regardless of the cause of the defective intestinal calcium absorption, and irrespective of where the primary insult occurred, this failure brings about increased dependence upon bone for calcium. Hence the vitamin D system may be important in the pathogenesis of postmenopausal osteoporosis in the following manner. At the onset of the menopause, bone may become more sensitive to mobilization by such factors as parathyroid hormone and $1,25\text{-}(OH)_2D_3$ (57). This could result, in turn, in suppression of parathyroid hormone secretion and $1,25\text{-}(OH)_2D_3$ production, which may lead to decreased intestinal calcium absorption. The decreased intestinal calcium absorption places a subtle but persistent reliance on calcium mobilization for maintaining plasma calcium concentration. This spiral then results in continual bone loss or negative calcium balance. Alternatively, the primary defect may lie in inappropriate response of $25\text{-}OH\text{-}D_3\text{-}1\text{-}alpha$-hydroxylase to parathyroid hormone. In such circumstances, one might expect either normal or higher than normal levels of parathyroid hormone and low levels of $1,25\text{-}(OH)_2D_3$. In any case, postmenopausal females treated with the 1-hydroxylated vitamins do show a response by eliciting an increased intestinal absorption or transport (Tables 1 and 2). Furthermore, balance studies carried out have indicated that for up to two years, as illustrated in Table 2, there is an improvement in calcium balance brought about by the administration of 0.5 mcg of $1,25\text{-}(OH)_2D_3$ daily to osteoporotic females (58, 59).

It is unknown whether this improvement in balance will bring about an improvement in bone mass. So far, there is no conclusive evidence for this point. In addition, it is unknown whether the active form of vitamin D can bring about new bone formation in sufficient quantities to increase bone mass of patients already suffering from osteoporosis.

Published data suggest that deficiency of $1,25\text{-}(OH)_2D_3$ is a significant factor in postmenopausal osteoporosis. Recent publications,

Table 1.   Responses to Treatment with 0.5 mcg/day 1, 25-(OH)$_2$Ds: Calcium Balance Studies (mean/day) at 6 months

Group	Time	Intake (mg)	Urine (mg)	% Net Abs	Balance (mg)
Placebo	Before	677	122	9.0	−36 mg
n=8	After	688	127	9.5	−43 mg
Treated	Before	759	116	6.5	−57 mg
n =8	After	745	190[a]	26.1[a]	+ 1 mg[b]

[a]Significance of change from treatment p <.01.
[b]p<.025 Calcium balance was more significantly related to calcium absorption (r = 0.86, p <.001) than to calcium intake (r = 0.56, p <.05). Reference: J. C. Gallagher, B. L. Riggs, and H. F. DeLuca, *Clin. Res.*, **27**, 366a, 1979.

Table 2.   Response to Treatment with 0.5 mcg/day 1, 25(OH)$_2$D$_3$

	Ca abs (%/6 hrs)	Ca Balance (mg/day)	Vo$^+$ (mg/day)	HyPro (mg/day)	BF (%)	BF (%)
Baseline	48	−50	221	26	1.8	8.3
6 Months	63[a]	+6[a]	167[a]	21[a]	2.5	5.7[a]
24 Months	65[a]	−30	257	22[a]	2.6	7.0

[a]Significance of change, p <0.05. n = 12. Reference: J. C. Gallagher, B. L. Riggs, and H. F. DeLuca, *Clin. Res.*, **28**, 777a, 1980.

including one from Japan (60), confirm the earlier observation of Riggs and DeLuca that serum levels of 1,25-(OH)$_2$D are subnormal in osteoporotic patients. Kumar et al. (61) have reported that plasma 1,25-(OH)$_2$D levels are elevated in early pregnancy, continue to increase throughout pregnancy, and remain elevated during lactation. It is noteworthy that this increase in 1,25-(OH)$_2$D levels coincides quite precisely with bone apposition in both mother and fetus as reported by Garn (62). Elevated levels have also been found in growing children (63) and in adult humans during healing of vitamin D deficiency osteomalacia (64). Therefore, convincing data are now available to show that 1,25-(OH)$_2$D levels are elevated during stages of human life when bone accretion takes place and, conversely, they are low when bone loss occurs or when mineralization of osteoid is impaired.

These findings suggest that Rocaltrol administration prevents bone mineral loss in postmenopausal women and justify additional studies to establish conclusively whether Rocaltrol is effective for the prevention and treatment of postmenopausal osteoporosis.

PHARMACOKINETICS

Single Dose

Plasma Levels and Kinetics.   The pharmacokinetics of calcitriol have been investigated in normal man. Gray et al. (65) studied a wide range of intravenously administered doses of tritium-radiolabeled calcitriol [^{3}H-1,25-(OH)$_2$D$_3$, 0.012–1.0 mcg] in seven healthy adults. The results of their study suggested that after a rapid loss of about 80% of the radio-activity from the plasma (half-life of about five minutes), the calcitriol levels decreased with a half-life of the order of ten hours. Only 14 ± 2% (range 10–16%) of the administered tritium remained in the plasma pool four hours after administration. The values were very similar for all subjects, despite an eightyfold variation in the administered dose. The calcitriol was rapidly metabolized; plasma metabolite profiles during the first four hours showed only 1,25-(OH)$_2$D$_3$; thereafter, detectable amounts of other metabolites were found. The six-day cumulative excretion of radioactive metabolites in the urine and feces averaged 16 ± 3% and 49 + 11%, respectively, of the administered dose. Compartmental analysis of the isotope data for the two subjects who received the two smallest doses of calcitriol (0.012 mcg) indicated that the rate of endogenous renal synthesis of 1,25-(OH)$_2$D$_3$ approximates 0.3–1.0 mcg/day.

Blumenthal et al. (66) gave single oral doses of either 0.25 mcg or 0.5 mcg of calcitriol (Rocaltrol) to six normal volunteers. Peak blood levels were reached three to six hours after administration and decreased with half-lives of three and five hours, respectively, for the 0.25 mcg and 0.5 mcg doses (66). The total serum 1,25-(OH)$_2$D$_3$ concentrations (endogenous plus exogenous) present 24 hours after administration of the 0.5 mcg dose of calcitriol matched the endogenous serum concentration prior to dosing.

Bell et al. (67) administered oral doses of 1 mcg and 5 mcg of calcitriol to 32 normal subjects and determined that the maximum concentration of serum 1,25-(OH)$_2$D$_3$ occurred at about three hours and that the concentration declined exponentially thereafter. The half-life was calculated to be between five and six hours and was independent of the dose. Baseline values [34.1 ± 1.4 pg/ml for 1,25-(OH)$_2$D$_3$] were observed at 24 hours. Based on these data, the turnover rate of 1,25-(OH)$_2$D$_3$ was estimated to be 0.5 mcg/day in one normal subject.

After oral administration of 4 mcg of calcitriol (Rocaltrol) to four normal volunteers, Mason et al. (68) found that peak serum concentrations of 1,25-(OH)$_2$D$_3$ were reached after four hours and had returned to baseline values 27 hours after administration. These results agreed with the data of Rosen et al. (69), who gave calcitriol orally (0.03–0.16 mcg/kg/ day) to three hypoparathyroid children and found raised serum concentrations four hours later, but not 16 hours later. Bell and Stern (70) administered calcitriol (Rocaltrol, 0.5–5 mcg/day) orally to two men with psuedohypoparathyroidism; they also observed basal values for serum 1,25-$(OH)_2D_3$ concentrations 24 hours after the last dose, except when the subjects had been hypercalcemic.

In a more recent study by Seeman et al. (71) 14 healthy control subjects received tracer doses (2.6–7.7 ng) of ^{3}H-1,25-$(OH)_2D_3$ in 2 ml propylene glycol as a single bolus intravenous injection. Approximately 30% of the administered tritium remained in the plasma pool ten minutes after the injection, and only about 16% remained at four hours. Chromatography of pooled plasma samples from time points 0 to 240 minutes showed only a single peak of radioactivity that cochromatographed with the 1,25-$(OH)_2D_3$ standard. By using a three-compartmental analysis model, the metabolic clearance rate was calculated to be 31 ± 4 ml/min and the endogenous production rate to be 1.5 ± 0.2 mcg/day, which was similar to the rate reported by Gray et al. (65). The six-day cumulative excretion of radioactivity from the body was 54 ± 6% of the administered dose in the stool and 14 ± 2% in the urine.

In a related study by Wiesner et al. (72) seven normal male subjects received a single bolus intravenous injection of 10 ng (tracer dose) of ^{3}H-1,25-$(OH)_2D_3$ in 1 ml of propylene glycol. Within 6.5 min, 50% of the administered dose was removed from the plasma; thereafter, the rate of decrease was slower, with 17% of the labeled dose remaining at six hours. Again, a three-compartment model was used to interpret the data, and the half-life of the third component of the ^{3}H-1,25-$(OH)_2D_3$ decay curve was 690 minutes, in accord with the data of Gray et al. (65) and Seeman et al. (71) on the disappearance of radioactivity from the circulation. Plasma concentrations were within the normal range.

In another recent study, four normal subjects received an oral dose of 2 mcg of calcitriol (73). Plasma levels of 1,25-$(OH)_2D_3$ (endogenous plus exogenous) were increased by 250 pmol/l (104 pg/ml), which was 100 pmol/l (41 pg/ml) above the normal range; the peak concentration occurred six hours after administration of the dose. At 22 hours, the plasma concentration was 125 pmol/l (52 pg/ml) above the basal concentration; by 46 hours, it had returned to basal values.

Enterohepatic Circulation.   In the study done by Wiesner et al. (72) the seven subjects were intubated with a triple-lumen nasoduodenal tube.

Analysis of samples taken from the duodenums of five subjects showed that, within 30 minutes of administration of ^{3}H-1,25-(OH)$_2$D$_3$, polar metabolites of 1,25-(OH)$_2$D$_3$ are excreted in the duodenum via the bile. The doses of calcitriol used in these experiments were small (10 ng). The excretion in the bile occurred at a constant rate, with a cumulative mean of 15.6% of the injected dose appearing in the duodenum within six hours. If this were to continue at the same rate, 62.4% of the injected dose would appear in the duodenum within 24 hours. However, only 27% and 7.5% of the injected dose appeared in the feces and urine, respectively, at 24 hours. In the other two subjects, biliary radioactivity was sampled at two sites separated by a distance of 40 cm; analysis of the samples indicated a 24.8% decrease in radioactivity over this segment of bowel. The authors concluded that products of 1,25-(OH)$_2$D$_3$ are excreted in normal human bile; and that, furthermore, these products are reabsorbed as such or as free 1,25-(OH)$_2$D$_3$ in the intestine and reexcreted as polar products in the bile, which suggests that there is an enterohepatic circulation of the products of 1,25-(OH)$_2$D$_3$ in normal man.

Multiple Dose

Gray et al. (74) studied the effects of chronic (seven day) oral calcitriol on plasma 1,25-(OH)$_2$D levels in six healthy men eating constant normal-calcium (19 + 3 mmol/day) and low calcium (4.2 ± 0.4 mmol/day) diets. Each of two subjects (one eating a low-calcium and one eating a normal-calcium diet) received 0.25, 0.5, or 0.75 mcg of calcitriol, four times a day, six hours apart; blood was sampled two, four, and six hours after dosing (at 2000, 1600, and 0600 hours, respectively). Plasma levels of 1,25-(OH)$_2$D were not dependent on dietary calcium levels. Table 3 shows the average 1,25-(OH)$_2$D levels for the men.

Table 3. Serum Levels of 1,25-(OH)$_2$D pmol/ml(pg/ml) Following Calcitriol Administration Every Six Hours

Hours After Previous Dose	0.25 mcg	0.5 mcg	0.75 mcg
2	124 (51.7)	172 (71.7)	170 (70.8)
4	126 (52.5)	198 (82.5)	221 (92.1)
6	115 (47.9)	172 (71.7)	208 (86.7)

The authors concluded that a new steady state was achieved and that, during calcitriol administration, serum calcitriol levels and the changes from control in serum calcitriol best fit a correlation with the log of the dose of calcitriol administered. They also stated that if the assumption is made that the effects of renal calcitriol synthesis on serum $1,25\text{-}(OH)_2D$ levels are quantitatively similar to the observed effects of oral calcitriol on such serum levels, the estimated endogenous renal calcitriol synthesis rate (based on these relationships, control calcitriol levels, and body weight) is about 1.7 nmol/day or 0.7 mcg/day, a value consistent with their previous estimate (65), which was based on the disappearance of injected $^3H\text{-}1,25\text{-}(OH)_2D_3$.

Bryce et al. (75) and Coburn et al. (76) carried out a study to determine whether there is an accumulation of calcitriol, as measured in blood levels, in normal humans receiving repeated doses of the drug. Six normal volunteers received calcitriol (Rocaltrol) in three different oral dosage regimens, each lasting one week: (1) 0.5 mcg once a day, (2) 0.25 mcg twice a day, 12 hours apart, and (3) 0.5 mcg twice a day, 12 hours apart. These doses are comparable to the magnitude of the turnover rate of $1,25\text{-}(OH)_2D_3$ (0.5 mcg/day) estimated by Bell et al. (67) and the endogenous synthesis rates estimated by Gray et al. (65) (0.3–1.0 mcg/day) and Seeman et al. (71) (1.5 ± 0.2 mcg/day). In most instances, the serum $1,25\text{-}(OH)_2D_3$ levels were statistically significantly elevated four hours after dosing, when compared to the predosing fasted levels (76). With all three regimens, a dose-related biological response was observed in the form of an increase in the daily urinary calcium excretion, despite only modest, but in some cases statistically significant, increases in circulating $1,25\text{-}(OH)_2D_3$. The 0.5 mcg dose caused a greater increase in urinary calcium excretion when divided into two 0.25 mcg doses given 12 hours apart, indicating that effective serum levels were maintained for a longer time with the two doses than with the single 0.5 mcg dose. No episodes of hypercalcemia occurred. There were no changes in the serum levels or in the urinary excretion of creatinine, phosphate, or magnesium throughout the course of the study.

In a further study by Coburn et al. (76) 14 volunteers received the following doses of calcitriol (Rocaltrol) twice a day (every 12 hours) for periods of 14 days with intervening control periods of 14 days: 0.25 mcg, 0.5 mcg, and 1.0 mcg. As in the previous studies (75, 76), a dose-related biological response was seen in the form of increased urinary calcium excretion. The mean response of urinary calcium to 0.25 mcg was not statistically significant; the mean response to 0.5 mcg was significant ($p < 0.05$) and was greater than that to 0.25 mcg. However, with the 1.0 mcg dose, while the increase was greater when compared to control

($p < 0.001$), the increase was not statistically significantly different from the value at 0.5 mcg, suggesting that maximal stimulation had been attained at a dose of less than 1.0 mcg. These changes in calcium excretion occurred with relatively modest, but statistically significant increases in serum 1,25-$(OH)_2D_3$ levels (57 ± 4 pg/ml vs. a control value of 39 ± 4, $p < 0.01$, for 0.5 mcg and 63 ± 5 pg/ml vs. 46 ± 3, $p < 0.01$, for 1.0 mcg). More important, these changes occurred without concomitant increases in the urinary excretion of hydroxyproline, suggesting a dietary origin of the excreted calcium rather than increased bone resorption.

The two higher doses of calcitriol also resulted in statistically significantly increased serum levels of 1,25-$(OH)_2D_3$ four hours after administration, when compared to the levels just prior to administration. The steady-state serum levels that resulted from the administration of the 0.5 mcg and 1.0 mcg doses both declined to basal values on cessation of drug, with a half-life of 3.5 hours. This value agreed with the values determined in other studies done with similar materials and assays (66–68, 75) and demonstrated that the decay rate from an elevated steady state (14 days of treatment) was comparable with that following the peak level of a single dose.

No episodes of hypercalcemia were seen at any time throughout the study. Although there were slight, statistically significant increases in serum phosphate at the 1.0 mcg dose ($p < 0.01$) and statistically significant decreases ($p < 0.01$) in serum magnesium at both the 0.25 mcg and 1.0 mcg doses, the decreases were judged not dose related and were not regarded as clinically significant. No statistically significant changes were recorded in the urinary excretions of phosphate, creatinine, or hydroxyproline throughout the study; the statistically significant decrease ($p < 0.05$) in urinary sodium was judged not dose related. No other changes in laboratory values were observed. With the exception of these slight changes, the consistent absence of changes demonstrates that calcitriol administration did not impair the normal mechanisms for mineral homeostasis or renal function.

Early Study

The initial study of the pharmacokinetics of calcitriol had been done by Mawer et al. (78), who used radiolabeled calcitriol. The radiolabeled calcitriol had been prepared by incubation of tritiated 25-OH-D_3 with homogenates of kidneys from vitamin D deficient chicks. The results of this study had suggested a distribution half-life of 14 hours and an elimination half-life of 81 hours.

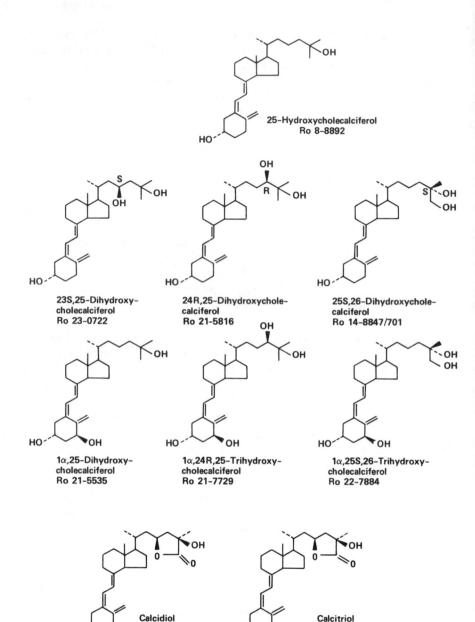

Figure 5. Structures and names of various natural metabolites of vitamin D$_3$ which have been chemically synthesized.

Summary of Pharmacokinetic Data

With the synthesis of larger amounts of analytically pure calcitriol and with the development of a calcitriol (Rocaltrol) and improved assays, better controlled studies of calcitriol have been possible. The recent experiments have shown much shorter elimination half-lives (3–10 hours) for calcitriol (66–68, 75, 77). Although some variability has been shown in these later studies, it is certain that the half-life is not in the order of 80 hours as first reported (78), since serum concentrations of $1,25\text{-}(OH)_2D_3$ have returned to basal values by 16 to 27 hours after administration of the last dose of calcitriol (66–70, 75–77).

THE FUTURE

Recently discovered metabolites of vitamin D (79) (Figure 5) and a number of synthetic analogs (80) (Figures 6–8) hold promise with regard to greater potency and fewer side effects. Some may be useful in the treatment of nephrolithiasis, primary hyperparathyroidism, hypercalcemia

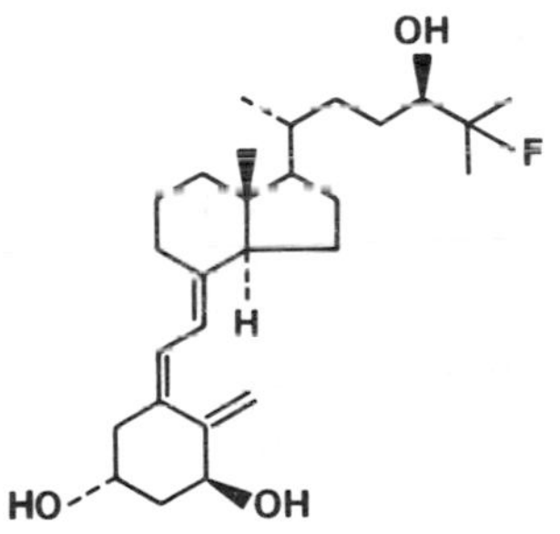

Figure 6. Structure of 1-alpha-24-$(OH)_2$-25-F-D_3.

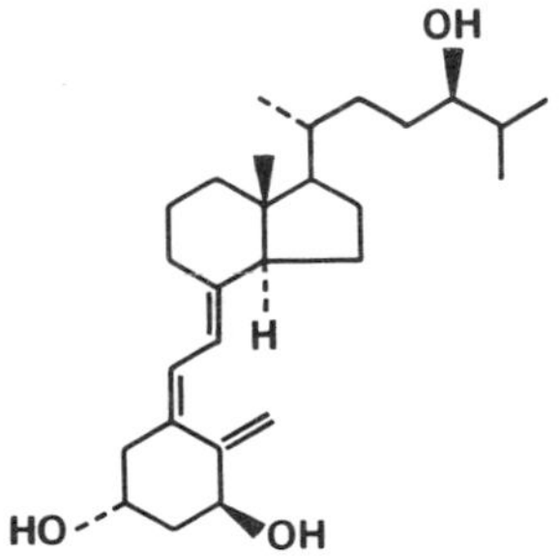

Figure 7. Structure of 1-alpha-24-$(OH)_2$-D_3.

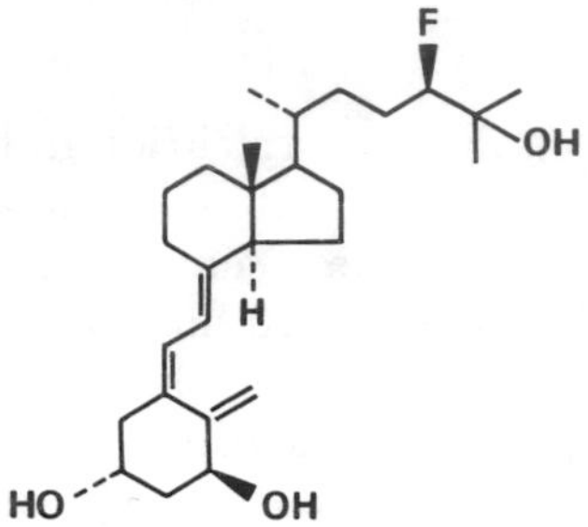

Figure 8.   Structure of 1-alpha-25(OH)$_2$-24R-F-D$_3$.

associated with such diseases as Boeck's sarcoidoses, and a variety of other diseases associated with bone and calcium-phosphorus homeostasis.

REFERENCES

1. H. F. DeLuca, *Nutr. Rev.*, **37,** 161 (1979).
2. H. F. DeLuca, *Nutr. Rev.*, **38,** 169 (1980).
3. M. R. Haussler and T. A. McCain, *N. Engl. J. Med.*, **297,** 974 and 1041 (1977).
4. E. Kodicek, *Lancet*, **1,** 325 (1974).
5. H. F. DeLuca, *Curr. Med. Res. Opin.*, **7**(5), 279 (1981).
6. R. P. Esvelt, H. K. Schnoes, and H. F. DeLuca, *Arch. Biochem. Biophys.*, 188, 282–286, (1978).
7. M. F. Holick, N. M. Richtand, S. C. McNeill, S. A. Holick, J. E. Frommer, J. W. Henley, and J. T. Potts, Jr., *Biochemistry*, **18,** 1003 (1979).
8. M. Bhattacharyya and H. F. DeLuca, *Arch. Biochem. Biophys.*, **160,** 58 (1974).
9. T. C. Madhok and H. F. DeLuca, *Biochem. J.*, **184,** 491–499, (1979).
10. P. S. Yoon and H. F. DeLuca, *Arch. Biochem. Biophys.*, **203,** 529 (1980).
11. I. Björkhem and I. Holmberg, *J. Biol. Chem.*, **253,** 842 (1978).
12. J. I. Pedersen, I. Holmberg, and I. Björkhem, *F.E.B.S. Lett.*, **98,** 394 (1979).
13. M. H. Bhattacharyya and H. F. DeLuca, *J. Biol. Chem.*, **248,** 2969 (1973).
14. M. H. Bhattacharyya and H. F. DeLuca, *Biochem. Biophys. Res. Commun.*, **59,** 734 (1974).
15. G. Tucker, III, R. E. Gagnon, and M. R. Haussler, *Arch. Biochem. Biophys.*, **155,** 47 (1973).
16. E. B. Olsen, Jr., J. C. Knuston, M. H. Bhattacharyya, and H. F. DeLuca, *J. Clin. Invest.*, **57,** 1213 (1976).
17. G. Ponchon, A. L. Kennan, and H. F. DeLuca, *J. Clin. Invest.*, **48,** 2032 (1969).
18. J. G. Ghazarian and H. F. DeLuca, *Arch. Biochem. Biophys.*, **160,** 63 (1974).
19. J. G. Ghazarian, C. R. Jefcoate, J. C. Knutson, W. H. Orme-Johnson, and H. F. DeLuca, *J. Biol. Chem.*, **249,** 3026 (1974).

20. R. W. Gray, J. L. Omdahl, J. G. Ghazarian, and H. F. DeLuca, *J. Biol. Chem.*, **247**, 7528 (1972).

21. M. Garabedian, Y. Tanaka, M. F. Holick, and H. F. DeLuca, *Endocrinology*, **94**, 1022 (1974).

22. I. T. Boyle, L. Miravet, R. W. Gray, M. F. Holick, and H. F. DeLuca, *Endocrinology*, **90**, 605 (1972).

23. M. F. Holick, M. Garabedian, and H. F. DeLuca, *Science*, **176**, 1146 (1972).

24. M. Garabedian, M. T. Corvol, T. M. Nguyen, and S. Balsan, *Ann. Biol. Anim. Biochem. Biophys.*, **18**, 175 (1978).

25. M. F. Holick, H. K. Schnoes, H. F. DeLuca, R. W. Gray, I. T. Boyle, and T. Suda, *Biochemistry*, **11**, 4251 (1972).

26. R. Kumar, H. K. Schnoes and H. F. DeLuca, *J. Biol. Chem.*, **253**, 3804 (1978).

27. D. Goodwin, D. Noff, and S. Edelstein, *Nature*, **276**, 517 (1978).

28. H. Rasmussen and P. Bordier, *Metab. Bone Dis. Rel. Res.*, **1**, 7 (1978).

29. M. Garabedian, M. Lieberherr, T. M. Nguyen, M. T. Corvol, M. B. Dubois, and S. Balsan, *Clin. Orthop.*, **135**, 241 (1978).

30. H. L. Henry and A. W. Norman, *Science*, **201**, 835 (1978).

31. S. C. Miller, B. P. Halloran, H. F. DeLuca, and W. S. S. Jee, *Calcif. Tissue Int.* (1980), In press.

32. R. Nicolaysen, N. Eeg-Larsen, and O. J. Malm, *Physiol. Rev.*, **33**, 424 (1953).

33. S. Okamoto, Y. Tanaka, H. F. DeLuca, S. Yamada, and H. Takayama, *Arch. Biochem. Biophys.*, **205**, (1980). In press.

34. Y. Tanaka, H. F. DeLuca, Y. Kobayashi, T. Taguchi, N. Ikekawa, and M. Morisaki, *J. Biol. Chem.*, **254**, 7163 (1979).

35. Y. Tanaka, J. K. Wichmann, H. E. Paaren, H. K. Schnoes, and H. F. DeLuca, *Proc. Natl. Acad. Sci. U.S.A.*, (1980), In press.

36. J. K. Wichmann, H. F. DeLuca, H. K. Schnoes, R. L. Horst, R. M. Shepard, and N. A. Jorgensen, *Biochemistry*, **18**, 4775 (1979).

37. Y. Tanaka, R. M. Shepard, H. F. DeLuca, and H. K. Schnoes, *Biochem. Biophys. Res. Commun.*, **83**, 7 (1978).

38. I. T. Boyle, R. W. Gray, and H. F. DeLuca, *Proc. Natl. Acad. Sci. U.S.A.*, **68**, 2131 (1971).

39. M. Garabedian, M. F. Holick, H. F. DeLuca, and I. T. Boyle, *Proc. Natl. Acad. Sci. U.S.A.*, **69**, 1673 (1972).

40. D. R. Fraser and E. Kodicek, *Nature New Biol.*, **241**, 163 (1973).

41. C. R. Kleeman, D. Bernstein, R. Rockney, J. T. Dowling, and M. H. Maxwell, "Studies on Renal Clearance of Diffusible Calcium and the Role of the Parathyroid Glands in its Regulation," in R. O. Greep and R. V. Talmage, Eds., *The Parathyroids*, Thomas, Springfield, Ill., 1961, p. 353.

42. R. A. L. Sutton and J. H. Dirks, *Fed. Proc.*, **37**, 2112 (1978).

43. Y. Tanaka and H. F. DeLuca, *Arch. Biochem. Biophys.*, **154**, 566 (1973).

44. Y. Tanaka, R. S. Lorenc, and H. F. DeLuca, *Arch. Biochem. Biophys.*, **171**, 521 (1975).

45. D. J. Brown, E. Spanos, and I. MacIntyre, *Br. Med. J.*, **2**, 277 (1980).

46. S. N. Baksi and A. D. Kenny, *Endocrinology*, **101**, 1216 (1977).

47. Y. Tanaka, L. Castillo, M. J. Wineland, and H. F. DeLuca, *Endocrinology*, **103**, 2035 (1978).

48. H. L. Henry, *J. Biol. Chem.*, **254**, 2722 (1979).

49. U. Trechsel, J. P. Bonjour, and H. Fleisch, *J. Clin. Invest.*, **64**, 206 (1979).

50. Y. Tanaka, B. Halloran, H. K. Schnoes, and H. F. DeLuca, *Proc. Natl. Acad. Sci. U.S.A.*, **76**, 5033 (1979).

51. C. Crilly, A. Horsman, D. H. Marshall, and B. E. C. Nordin, *Aust. N.Z.J. Med.*, **9**, 24 (1979).

52. H. F. DeLuca, H. M. Frost, W. S. S. Jee, C. C. Johnston, and A. M. Parfitt, Eds., *Osteoporosis: Recent Advances in Pathogenesis and Treatment*, University Park Press, Baltimore, 1980.

53. R. P. Heaney, "Vitamin D and Osteoporosis," in A. W. Horman, K. Scheafer, J. W. Coburn, H. F. DeLuca, H. G. Grigoleit and D. von Herrath, Eds., *Vitamin D: Biochemical, Chemical and Clinical Aspects Related to Calcium Metabolism*, Walter de Gruyter, Berlin, 1977, p. 627.

54. R. L. Horst, H. F. DeLuca, and N. A. Jorgensen, *Metab. Bone Dis. Rel. Res.*, **1**, 29 (1978).

55. J. C. Gallagher, B. L. Riggs, J. Eisman, S. Arnaud, and H. F. DeLuca, *Clin. Res.*, **24**, 360A (1976).

56. H. F. DeLuca, "Vitamin D," in H. F. DeLuca, Ed. *The Fat-Soluble Vitamins*, Plenum, New York, 1978, p. 69.

57. B. L. Riggs, J. Jowsey, P. J. Kelly, and C. D. Arnaud, *Isr. J. Med. Sci.*, **12**, 615 (1976).

58. J. C. Gallagher, B. L. Riggs, J. Eisman, A. Hamstra, S. B. Arnaud, and H. F. DeLuca, *J. Clin. Invest.*, **64**, 729 (1979).

59. B. L. Riggs, J. C. Gallagher, and H. F. DeLuca, "Osteoporosis and Age-related Osteopenia: Evaluation of Possible Role of Vitamin D Endocrine System in Pathogenesis of Impaired Intestinal Calcium Absorption," in A. W. Norman, K. Schaefer, D.V. Herrath, H. G. Grigoleit, J. W. Coburn, H. F. DeLuca, E. B. Mawer, and T. Suda, Eds., *Vitamin D: Basic Research and Its Clinical Application*, Walter de Gruyter, Berlin, 1979, p. 107.

60. K. Okano, R. Nakai, and M. Haraswa, *Endocrinol. Japan*, S. R. No. **1**, 23 (1979).

61. R. Kumar, W. R. Cohen, P. Silva, and F. H. Epstein, *J. Clin. Invest.*, **63**, 342 (1979).

62. S. M. Garn, *The Earlier Gain and the Later Loss of Cortical Bone*, Springfield, Ill., Charles C. Thomas, 1970.

63. R. W. Chesney, J. Rosen, A. Hamstra, and H. F. DeLuca, *Am. J. Dis. Children*, **134**, 135 (1980).

64. S. E. Papapoules, L. J. Fraher, T. L. Clemens, J. Gleed, and J. C. H. O'Riordan, *Lancet*, **2**, 612 (1980).

65. R. W. Gray, A. E. Caldas, D. R. Wilz, J. Lemann, Jr., G. A. Smith, and H. F. DeLuca, *J. Clin. Endocrinol. Metab.*, **46**, 756 (1978).

66. H. P. Blumenthal, et al., personal communication, (1980).

67. N. H. Bell, P. C. Schaefer, and R. Goldsmith, *Calcif. Tissue Int.*, **28**, 172 (1979).

68. R. S. Mason, D. Lissner, S. Posen, and A. W. Norman, *Br. Med. J.*, **280**, 449 (1980).

69. J. F. Rosen, A. R. Fleischman, L. Finberg, J. Eisman, and H. F. DeLuca, *J. Clin. Endocrinol. Metab.*, **45**, 457 (1977).

70. N. H. Bell and P. H. Stern, *N. Engl. J. Med.*, **298**, 1241 (1978).

71. E. Seeman, R. Kumar, G. G. Hunder, M. Scott, H. Heath, III, and B. L. Riggs, *J. Clin. Invest.*, **66**, 664 (1980).

72. R. H. Wiesner, R. Kumar, E. Seeman, and V. L. W. Go, *J. Lab. Clin. Med.*, **96**, 1094 (1980).

73. W. B. Brown, M. Peacock, G. A. Taylor, A. Davies, and P. J. Heyburn, *J. Endocrinol.*, **87**, 16P (1980).

74. R. W. Gray, N. D. Adams, and J. Lemann, Jr., *Clin. Res.*, **28**, 739A (1980).

75. G. F. Bryce, et al., personal communication (1980).

76. J. W. Coburn, G. F. Bryce, B. S. Levine, J. P. Mallon, S. N. Winkler, and O. N. Miller, *Clin. Res.*, **28**, 79A (1980).

77. G. F. Bryce, et al., personal communication (1980).

78. E. B. Mawer, J. Backhouse, M. Davies, L. F. Hill, and C. M. Taylor, *Lancet* **1**, 1203 (1976).

79. H. F. DeLuca, et al., personal communication.

80. M. Uskokovic and A. Boris, personal communication.

4

Alcohol, Protein Nutrition, and Liver Injury

CHARLES S. LIEBER

Alcohol Research and Treatment Center, Bronx VA Medical Center and Mount Sinai School of Medicine (CUNY), New York, New York

Alcohol is both a food and a drug. Alcohol is rich in energy and in many societies, alcoholic beverages are considered part of the basic food supply. Alcohol is also consumed for its mood-altering effects and therefore plays the role of a psychoactive drug. Under both circumstances, large intake of alcohol results in various toxic effects. Hardly any tissue in the body escapes the toxicity of alcohol. Tissues most strikingly affected are the brain and the liver. Possible interrelationships between alcoholism, malnutrition, and liver disease are complex: alcoholism commonly causes both malnutrition and liver disease, and liver dysfunction may be engendered by malnutrition per se. Moreover, about thirty years ago, some emphasis was given to the possibility that malnutrition may promote alcoholism. More recently, however, that notion has lost its appeal. Indeed, it is now generally accepted that vitamin therapy does not reduce addiction to alcohol in man. Several neurological complications of alcoholism, such as polyneuropathy and Wernicke's syndrome, once thought to be due to a direct toxic effect of alcohol, have now clearly been recognized as vitamin deficiencies resulting primarily from an inadequate thiamine intake. A reverse trend of thought has occurred with regard to liver disease and associated metabolic disturbances of alcoholism. Whereas traditionally, the disorders affecting the liver have been attributed exclusively to nutritional deficiencies accompanying alcoholism, recent studies, summarized here, indicate that in addition to the role of dietary deficiencies, alcohol per se can be incriminated as a direct etiologic factor in the production of alcoholic liver disease. Moreover, secondary malnutrition has now come to the forefront with the demonstration that dietary deficiency is not the sole cause of malnutrition in the alcoholic but that alcohol has also some direct effects upon the gastrointestinal tract, resulting in maldigestion and malabsorption of essential nutrients as discussed in more detail elsewhere (1). This chapter will focus on damage produced in the liver. The early stages of liver injury are characterized by accumulation of excess fat in the liver, or fatty liver. When there is superimposed necrosis and inflammation, the term alcoholic hepatitis is used to characterize this more advanced phase. Finally, when extensive scarring develops, the ultimate and irreversible stage of cirrhosis is reached. Here we will focus on the pathogenesis of these complications, especially the interaction of the intrinsic toxicity of alcohol with severe nutritional disorders associated with alcoholism, particularly the deficiencies in protein and vitamins.

Chronic alcohol consumption does indeed therefore interfere with normal food digestion and absorption because of its well-known effects on gut and pancreas. Furthermore, alcohol, high in caloric values, displaces other foods in the diet. Each gram of ethanol provides 7.1 calories. Twelve ounces of an 86-proof beverage contain about 1200 calories, or approximately one-half the recommended daily dietary allowance for calories. But unlike regular food, alcoholic beverages contain few, if any, vitamins, minerals, protein, or other nutrients, and therefore the alcoholic's intake of these nutrients may readily become insufficient. Economic factors may also reduce consumption of nutrient-rich food, particularly those containing proteins. When these various states of malnutrition are superimposed on the intrinsic toxicity of alcohol, particularly severe damage may ensue.

PATHOGENESIS OF THE ALCOHOLIC FATTY LIVER

Etiologic Role of Ethanol

Until two decades ago the concept prevailed that malnutrition alone was responsible for the development of the alcoholic fatty liver. This notion was based largely on experimental work in rats given ethanol in drinking water (2). With this technique, ethanol consumption usually does not exceed 10–25% of the caloric intake of the animal. A comparable amount of alcohol, when given with an adequate diet, resulted in negligible ethanol levels in the blood (3). By incorporating ethanol in a totally liquid diet, the amount of ethanol consumed was increased to 36% of total calories, a proportion comparable to moderate alcohol intake in man. With these nutritionally adequate diets, isocaloric replacement of sucrose or other carbohydrate by ethanol consistently produces a fivefold to tenfold increase in hepatic triglycerides (3–6). It is noteworthy that isocaloric replacement of carbohydrate by fat instead of ethanol did not produce steatosis. Hepatic lipid accumulation developed progressively over the first month of alcohol administration and persisted thereafter for at least one year in the rat (6) and many years in the baboon (7–9). Moreover, individuals with a morphologically normal liver (with or without a history of alcoholism) developed a fatty liver when given ethanol in a variety of nondeficient diets as an isocaloric substitute for carbohydrates (3,4,10). This was evident both by morphological examination and by direct measurement of the lipid content of the liver biopsies, which revealed up to a twenty-fivefold rise in triglyceride concentration. Even with a high-protein, vitamin-supplemented diet, there was a significant increase in hepatic triglycerides, as measured in percutaneous biopsies (Figure 1). These studies, therefore, established the fact that even in the presence of an adequate diet ethanol can produce a fatty liver.

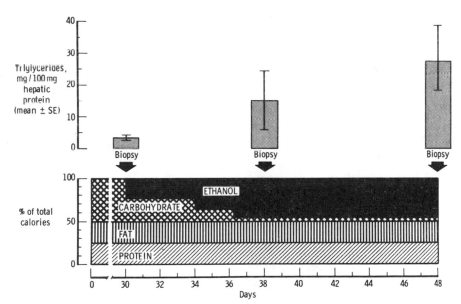

Figure 1. Effect of ethanol on hepatic triglycerides in five volunteers given a high-protein, low-fat diet. There was a striking increase in spite of the good diet (22).

The Influence of Dietary Factors

Role of Dietary Fat.   As discussed before, alcohol ingestion leads to the deposition of dietary fat in the liver. This observation prompted an investigation into the role of the amount and kind of dietary fat in the pathogenesis of alcohol-induced liver injury. Rats were given liquid diets containing a constant amount of ethanol (36% of energy), an adequate amount of protein for rodents (18% of total calories), and varying amounts of fat (Figure 2). In the 2% fat diet the only lipid given was linoleate, to avoid essential fatty acid deficiency. Reduction in dietary fat to a level of 25% (or less) of total calories was accompanied by a significant decrease in the steatosis induced by ethanol (6). These results obtained with alcohol differ from the fatty liver resulting from choline deficiency, the degree of which was found to be independent of the amount of dietary fat (11). The importance of dietary fat was confirmed in volunteers: for a given alcohol intake, much more steatosis developed

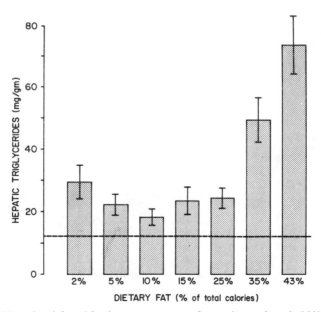

Figure 2.   Hepatic triglycerides in seven groups of rats given ethanol (36% of calories) with a diet normal in protein (18% of calories) but varying in fat content. Average hepatic triglyceride concentration in the control animals is indicated by a dotted line. A reduction of dietary fat decreased the capacity of alcohol to produce steatosis (6).

with diets of normal fat content than with low-fat diets (12). In addition to the amount, the chain length of the dietary fatty acid is also important for the degree of fat deposition in the liver. Replacement of dietary triglycerides containing long-chain fatty acids (LCT) by fat containing medium-chain fatty acids (MCT) reduces the capacity of alcohol to produce a fatty liver in rats (13). The propensity of medium-chain fatty acids to undergo oxidation rather than esterification probably explains this phenomenon (14).

Role of Protein and Lipotropic Factors (Choline and Methionine).   In growing rats, deficiencies in dietary protein and lipotropic factors (choline and methionine) can produce a fatty liver (2), whereas primates are far less susceptible to protein and lipotropic deficiency than rodents (15). Clinically, treatment with choline of patients suffering from alcoholic liver injury has been found to be ineffective in the face of continued alcohol abuse (16–19) and, experimentally, massive supplementation with choline failed to prevent the fatty liver produced by alcohol in volunteer subjects (20). This is not surprising, since unlike rat liver, human liver contains very little choline oxidase activity, which may explain the species differences with regard to choline deficiency. Thus, hepatic injury induced by choline deficiency appears to be primarily an experimental disease of rats, with little, if any, relevance to human alcoholic liver injury. Even in rats, massive choline supplementation failed to fully prevent the ethanol-induced lesion, whether alcohol was administered acutely (21) or chronically (13).

The effect of protein deficiency has not yet been clearly delineated in human adults. In children, protein deficiency leads to hepatic steatosis, one of the manifestations of kwashiorkor. In adolescent baboons, protein restriction to 7% of total calories did not result in conspicuous liver injury, even after 19 months, either by biochemical analysis or by light and electron microscopic examination. Significant steatosis was observed only when the protein intake was reduced to 4% of total calories (7). On the other hand, an excess of protein (25% of total calories, or 2.5 times the recommended amount) did not prevent ethanol from producing fat accumulation in human volunteers (Figure 1). Thus, in man, ethanol is capable of producing striking changes in liver lipids even in the presence of a protein-enriched diet. When protein deficiency is present, it may potentiate the effect of ethanol. In the rat, a combination of ethanol and a diet deficient in both protein and lipotropic factors leads to more pronounced hepatic steatosis than will either factor alone (23,24) (Figure 3). This potentiation is not unexpected, since increased lipoprotein secre-

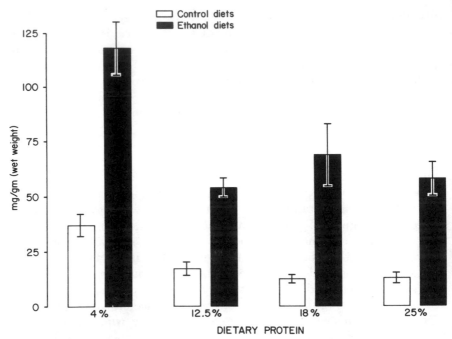

Figure 3.   Hepatic triglycerides in rats fed diets with normal fat content (35% of total calories), varying amounts of proteins, and either ethanol (36% of total calories) or isocaloric
carbohydrate (controls) (24).

tion offsets, in part, the alcohol-induced steatosis. Protein and/or choline
deficiency results in impaired lipoprotein secretion, which can be expected to markedly potentiate hepatic lipid accumulation secondary to
alcohol. In addition to its role as lipotrope, methionine may also act as a
cysteine and glutathione precursor, thereby affecting lipid peroxidation.

Origin of the Fatty Acids that are Deposited in the Alcoholic Fatty Liver and Mechanism for their Accumulation

Lipids that accumulate in the liver can originate from three main
sources: dietary lipids, which reach the bloodstream as chylomicrons;
adipose tissue lipids, which are transported to the liver as free fatty acids
(FFA); and lipids synthesized in the liver itself (Figure 4). These fatty
acids can accumulate in the liver because of a variety of metabolic disturbances (25). The five major mechanisms that have been proposed
are: (1) decreased lipid breakdown, including lipid oxidation in the liver,

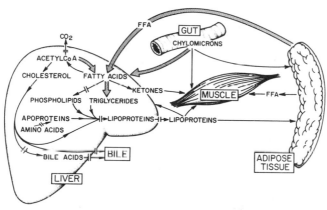

Figure 4. Possible mechanisms of fatty liver production through either increase (⟶) or decrease (⟶⊣ ⊢⟶) of lipid transport and metabolism (1).

(2) enhanced hepatic lipogenesis, (3) decreased hepatic release of lipoproteins, (4) increased mobilization of peripheral fat, and (5) enhanced hepatic uptake of circulating lipids. Depending on the experimental conditions, any of the three sources and the various mechanisms can be implicated.

Actually, peripheral fat mobilization is of little clinical relevance after chronic ethanol consumption. Under the latter conditions, the fatty acids deposited in the liver do not derive primarily from adipose tissue (12,26): after consumption of ethanol with lipid-containing diets, the fatty acids that accumulate in the liver are derived primarily from dietary fatty acids, whereas when ethanol is given with a low-fat diet, endogenously synthesized fatty acids are deposited in the liver (12,26,27). Some of these effects can be considered to be consequences of the metabolism of ethanol in the liver. Indeed, as discussed elsewhere (1), both decreased lipid oxidation and enhanced lipogenesis can be linked to ethanol oxidation and the associated increased generation of NADH (Figure 5).

In addition to the metabolic changes which are a direct consequence of the oxidation of ethanol, chronic ethanol abuse results in more persistent changes in the mitochondria. The striking structural changes of the mitochondria are associated with corresponding functional abnormalities, including depressed hepatic fatty acid oxidation.

Thus, the main event leading to the development of the alcoholic fatty liver can be summarized as follows: ethanol, which has an almost "obligatory" hepatic metabolism, replaces the fatty acids as a normal fuel

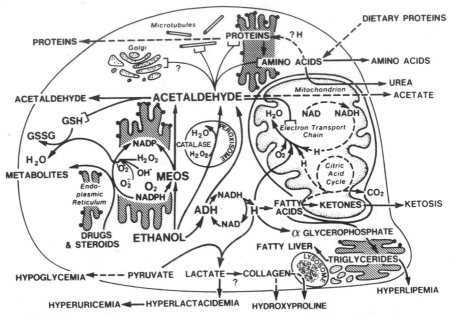

Figure 5. Oxidation of ethanol in the hepatocyte and link of the two metabolites (acetaldehyde and H) to disturbances in intermediary metabolism. NAD denotes nicotinamide adenine dinucleotide, NADP nicotinamide adenine dinucleotide phosphate, MEOS the microsomal ethanol oxidizing system, and ADH alcohol dehydrogenase. The broken lines indicate pathways that are depressed by ethanol. The symbol ——⊏⊐ denotes interference or binding by the metabolite (1).

for the hepatic mitochondria. This results in fatty acid accumulation directly, because of decreased lipid oxidation, and indirectly, because one way for the liver to dispose of excess hydrogen generated by ethanol oxidation is to synthesize more lipids. Fatty acids derived from adipose tissue accumulate in the liver only when very large amounts of ethanol are given. The lipids increase in the liver despite the fact that the transport mechanism via release of lipoproteins from the liver into the blood stream is stimulated by ethanol, at least during the initial state of intoxication. At one point, an equilibrium is reached between a lessening in lipid oxidation (due to progressive attenuation of redox change) and enhanced lipoprotein secretion. Lipids, then cease to accumulate further.

Later, with progressing liver injury, the hypersecretion of lipoprotein ceases and may actually fall below normal levels. At that stage, instead of offsetting, in part, the lipid accumulation, altered lipoprotein secretion may actually contribute to it and thereby aggravate fat accumulation and liver injury even further.

In addition to changes in carbohydrate and lipids, the abnormal redox state may also affect protein metabolism. Inhibition of protein synthesis has been observed after addition of ethanol to various preparations in vitro (28,29). In vivo, the acute effects of ethanol on protein synthesis have been less consistent than those described in vitro. No changes in the synthesis of total liver protein were found after administration of ethanol to well-fed naive rats (30). It would be of great interest to identify in vivo conditions that mimic the alterations of ethanol metabolism occurring in isolated liver preparations and that induce inhibitory effects of ethanol on protein synthesis. Indeed, under such conditions, the toxicity of ethanol should be greatly enhanced. One of these aggravating factors may be the hypoxia that normally prevails in the perivenular area of the liver and strikingly exaggerates the redox shift after ethanol (31).

AGGRAVATION OF HEPATOTOXICITY THROUGH MICROSOMAL "INDUCTION"

Chronic ethanol consumption results in proliferation of the membranes of the smooth endoplasmic reticulum, documented by subfractionation and chemical measurements in microsomes and by electron microscopy in animals and man (32,33). Proliferation is thought to be "adaptive," since it is associated with enhanced activity of the microsomal enzymes involved in lipoprotein production and thus may contribute to the increased capacity of the liver to secrete fat, as lipoproteins, into the bloodstream (34). A concomitant increase in drug-metabolizing enzymes explains the enhanced metabolic tolerance of patients with alcoholism to a variety of drugs. The activity of the microsomal ethanol-oxidizing system is also increased in these patients, and this increase may contribute to the accelerated rate of alcohol metabolism that occurs after chronic alcohol consumption. The latter may be viewed as the raison d'etre of the induction.

Although these microsomal changes can be interpreted as "adaptive" alterations secondary to "induction" after chronic ingestion of alcohol, some injurious consequences may also ensue. Indeed, accelerated ethanol metabolism results in enhanced production of acetaldehyde and exacerbation of its various toxic manifestations discussed subsequently, including enhanced peroxidation. The latter may also be promoted more directly through enhanced "free radical" formation by the induced microsomes. Similarly, increased microsomal activity may enhance the oxygen requirements, thereby aggravating whatever hypoxia may be present. Furthermore, some compounds acquire hepatotoxicity only after metabolism, or "activation," by the enzymes of the endoplasmic reticulum. One such compound is carbon tetrachloride, the hepatotoxicity of which is greatly increased after chronic alcohol consumption, at least partly because of enhanced activation by microsomes (35). It is likely that a similar mechanism increases susceptibility in these patients to the hepatotoxic actions of a variety of compounds in the environment, including many commonly used drugs, such as ioniazid and acetaminophen (36).

Miconutrients such as vitamins may also serve as substrates for the microsomes and the "induction" of the microsomes may therefore alter vitamin requirements and even affect the integrity of the liver. Indeed it has been found recently that alcoholics commonly have very low vitamin A levels in their livers (37). In experimental animals, ethanol administration was shown to depress hepatic vitamin A levels, even when administered with adequate diets (38) (Figure 6). When dietary vitamin A was virtually eliminated, the depletion rate of vitamin A endogenous hepatic storage was two to three times faster in ethanol-fed rats than in controls, possibly because of accelerated degradation of retinoic acid by the induced microsomes. In rats, severe vitamin A depletion was associated

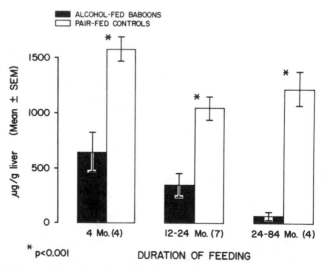

Figure 6. Effect of chronic ethanol feeding on hepatic vitamin A levels in baboons. Baboons were pair-fed ethanol (black bar) or control diet (white bar) and fasted for 12 hours before sampling. Ethanol was withdrawn 20 hours before sampling. Number of pairs is shown in parenthesis. Animals fed ethanol for 4–24 months showed hepatic steatosis, whereas fibrosis or cirrhosis was produced in the 24–84 months group (38).

with the appearance of multivesicular lysosomes (37). Such lesions were commonly seen in alcoholic patients with low hepatic A levels. Thus, vitamin A depletion may contribute to the liver lesions of the alcoholic. Vitamin A supplementation is sometimes used to correct the problems of night blindness and sexual dysfunctions of the alcoholic. Such therapy might be useful with regard to the liver pathology. The therapeutic use of vitamin A, however, is complicated by the facts that excessive amounts of vitamin A are known to be hepatotoxic and that the alcoholic may have an enhanced susceptibility to this effect (39). In control rats, amounts of vitamin A equivalent to those commonly used for the treatment of the alcoholic were found to be without significant effects on the liver, but in animals chronically fed alcohol, signs of toxicity developed, such as striking morphologic and functional alterations of the mitochondria (39) (Figure 7). Enhanced toxicity was not associated with an increased vitamin A level in the liver. In fact, bcause (as mentioned before) alcohol administration tends to decrease vitamin A levels in the liver, even after vitamin A supplementation alcohol-fed animals had vitamin A levels in the liver that were not higher than normal values. Nevertheless, toxicity developed. One possible explanation, still to be proven, is that vitamin A toxicity may be mediated at least in part by the enhanced production of a toxic metabolite, as in the case of xenobiotic agents. Thus the toxicity could be related to the induction of the enzymes of the endoplasmic reticulum after chronic ethanol consumption.

There are a number of other effects of microsomal induction discussed in detail elsewhere (1); They involve predominantly endocrine functions and overall energy metabolism of the body (40).

EFFECTS OF ACETALDEHYDE INCLUDING ITS INTERACTION WITH AMINO ACIDS AND PROTEINS

Acetaldehyde is the first major "specific" oxidation product of ethanol, whether the ethanol is oxidized by the classic alcohol dehydrogenase of the cytosol or by the more recently described microsomal system.

Acetaldehyde is a very reactive compound. It was found capable of "binding" to proteins, an effect enhanced by chronic ethanol consumption (41). Covalent binding of "active" metabolites has been incriminated in the hepatotoxicity of many drugs; this could also pertain to acetaldehyde, the active metabolite of ethanol.

Little was known about blood acetaldehyde levels after alcohol consumption until Korsten et al. (42) demonstrated a difference in blood acetaldehyde level between alcoholic and nonalcoholic subjects after comparable ethanol challenges. The mean acetaldehyde plateau level

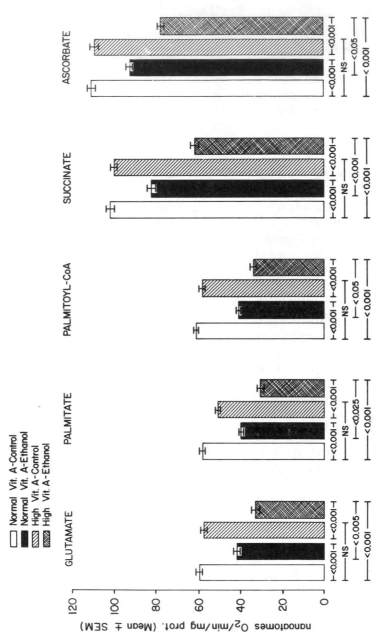

Figure 7. Effect of high vitamin A and/or chronic ethanol feeding on oxygen consumption of isolated mitochondria in state-3 respiration. High vitamin A by itself had no effect, whereas feeding of ethanol with a normal diet resulted in a depression of the oxygen consumption with all substrates; this effect was potentiated by high vitamin A. For each group the values are given as mean ± SEM of 11 pairs of animals (39).

was significantly higher in alcoholic than in nonalcoholic subjects. Recent methodologic advances have revealed that the concentration of acetaldehyde is lower than the levels previously reported. However, even at the lower level, blood acetaldehyde is increased after chronic alcohol consumption (43,44), probably reflecting increased production coupled with decreased disposition. Decreased catabolism is possibly due to alcohol-induced liver damage. Indeed, early structural changes are induced by alcohol in liver organelles, including the mitochondria (32,33). In rats fed ethanol chronically, Hasumura et al. (45) found that the liver mitochondria had a significantly reduced capacity to oxidize acetaldehyde.

The reduction of acetaldehyde metabolism associated with an enhanced production rate of acetaldehyde might result in the accumulation of acetaldehyde in the liver as well as in the blood. The enhanced acetaldehyde may in turn explain a number of ethanol-related complications.

Structural and Functional Alterations of the Mitochondria

Studies with the electron microscope have revealed striking morphologic alterations, including swelling and abnormal cristae, in the liver mitochondria of alcoholics. Controlled studies in animals and man (10,32,33,46) have shown that these changes are caused by alcohol itself, rather than by other factors, such as a poor diet. These structural abnormalities are associated with functional impairments, especially decreased oxidation of fatty acids and of a variety of other substrates, including acetaldehyde (45). Mitochondria of alcohol-fed animals have a reduction in cytochrome a and b content (47,48) and in succinic dehydrogenase activity (48,49). The respiratory capacity of the mitochondria was found to be depressed (50–53) using pyruvate, succinate, and acetaldehyde as substrates. Mg^{2+} stimulated ATPase activity may be either decreased or normal, depending on experimental conditions (54). Use of albumin devoid of free fatty acids in vitro and feeding of a high-protein, low-carbohydrate diet in vivo was also found to prevent the ethanol-induced changes (55). These are, however, highly artificial conditions, and as pointed out before, in human volunteers given ethanol, mitochondrial lesions developed even in the presence of a high-protein, low-fat diet (10).

Oxidative phosphorylation was found to be altered (56). It is noteworthy that high concentrations of acetaldehyde, the product of ethanol metabolism, mimic the defects produced by chronic ethanol consumption on oxidative phosphorylation (57). One may wonder to what extent chronic exposure to acetaldehyde is the cause for the defect observed after chronic ethanol consumption. As has been pointed out, alcoholics may exhibit higher acetaldehyde levels than nonalcoholics for a given ethanol load and blood level. It is therefore reasonable to speculate that exposure to high acetaldehyde levels may in turn affect mitochondrial function.

After chronic alcohol consumption, the liver mitochondria are unusually susceptible to the toxic effects of acetaldehyde, and a variety of important mitochondrial functions, such as fatty acid oxidation, are depressed, even in the presence of relatively low acetaldehyde concentrations.

Promotion of Lipid Peroxidation; Interaction with Cysteine and Glutathione

Aldehydes react quite readily with mercaptans, and L-cysteine could complex with acetaldehyde to form a hemiacetal. It has been suggested that such a complex may be a nontoxic detoxification product, since cysteine was reported to protect against death from acetaldehyde toxicity in vivo (58). Cysteine, in vitro, afforded protection against the depression of CO_2 production from palmitate, octanoate, and ketoglutarate by acetaldehyde (59). On the other hand, cysteine is one of the three amino acids that constitute glutathione. Binding of acetaldehyde with cysteine and/or glutathione may contribute to a depression of liver glutathione (60). Glutathione offers one of the mechanisms for the scavenging of toxic free radicals; a severe reduction in glutatione favors peroxidation (61), and the damage may possible be compounded by the increased generation of active radicals by the "induced" microsomes following chronic ethanol consumption, as illustrated in Figure 8. It is well known that the microsomal pathway, which requires O_2 and NADPH, is capable of generating lipid peroxides. Enhanced lipid peroxidation, possibly mediated by acetaldehyde (62), has been proposed as a mechanism for ethanol-induced fatty liver (63), but its role has been controversial (64–67). Theoretically, increased activity of microsomal NADPH oxidase following ethanol consumption (68,69) could result in enhanced H_2O_2 production, thereby also favoring lipid peroxidation.

In any event, it was found that in naive rats, very large amounts of ethanol (5–6g/kg) are required to produce lipid peroxidation (63,70), whereas a smaller dose (3g/kg) had no effect (60). By contrast, after chronic ethanol administration to the rat, even the smaller dose of etha-

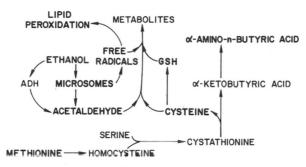

Figure 8. Hypothetical link between accelerated acetaldehyde production, increased free radical generation by the "induced" microsomes, and enhanced lipid peroxidation and possibly increased AANB (α-amino n butyric acid) production (105).

nol administered acutely induced liver peroxidation and this effect could be prevented, at least in part, by the administration of methionine, a precursor of glutathione (60). The ethanol-induced lipid peroxidation was even more striking in the baboon: administration of relatively small doses of ethanol (1–2g/kg) after five to six hours produced lipid peroxidation and GSH depletion. In the baboon chronically fed alcohol (50% of total calories for one to four years), alcoholic liver disease, including cirrhosis in some, develops and such animals exhibit evidence of enhanced hepatic lipid peroxidation and GSH depletion. These changes were observed following an overnight withdrawal from ethanol and were exacerbated by the readministration of ethanol. It is tempting to speculate that the propensity of the baboon to develop more severe lesions than the rat after chronic ethanol consumption may in some way be related, at least in part, to the greater susceptibility to glutathione depletion and the initiation of lipid peroxidation. It is apparent, however, that glutathione depletion per se does not suffice to produce liver damage (71). As mentioned before, concomitant enhanced production of active radicals may be required, possibly resulting from the microsomal "induction."

Swelling of the Hepatocyte and Possible Relation to Microtubular Alterations and Necrosis

Two of the earliest and most conspicuous features of the hepatic damage produced by alcohol are the deposition of fat and the enlargement of the liver. This hepatomegaly was traditionally attributed to the accumulation of lipids. However, in animals fed alcohol-containing diets it was shown that lipids account for only half the increase in liver dry weight (72), while the other half is almost totally accounted for by an increase in proteins (73), possibly secondary to acetaldehyde-induced impairment of microtubular-mediated protein secretion. Indeed, microtubules are shortened and thickened (74). It is noteworthy that impairment of microtubules was found to affect hepatocellular transport of biliary lipids (75) and to be associated with engorgement of the Golgi (74). The increase in hepatic protein observed after ethanol feeding was not associated with changes in concentration (76), indicating that water was retained in proportion to the increase in protein. The mechanism of the water retention is not fully elucidated, but the rise in both protein and amino acids, plus a likely increase in associated small ions, could account osmotically for a large fraction of the water increase. The increases in lipid, protein, amino acid, water, and electrolytes result in increased size of the hepatocytes. The number of hepatocytes and the hepatic content of deoxyribonucleic acid (DNA) did not change after alcohol treatment and thus the hepatomegaly is entirely accounted for by the increased cell volume (73,76). There is also an increase in the number of hepatic mesenchymal cells after ethanol feeding (73), but this increase does not significantly contribute to the hepatomegaly. The swelling of the hepatocytes after chronic alcohol administration was found to be associated with a reduction of the intercellular space and with portal hypertension (77). One suspects that ballooning and associated gross distortion of the volume of the hepatocytes may result in severe impairment of key cellular functions. In alcohlic liver disease, the diameter of some cells not uncommonly is increased two to three times, and thereby volume is increased about fourfold to tenfold. One may wonder to what extent this type of cellular disorganization, with protein retention and ballooning, may promote progresion of the liver injury in the alcoholic. Indeed, there are other causes of protein retention in the liver, such as alpha$_1$ antitrypsin deficiency, associated with progression to fibrosis and cirrhosis. By analogy, one can assume that protein retention may in some way also favor progression of liver disease in the alcoholic.

DISORDERS OF COLLAGEN METABOLISM AND PRODUCTION OF CIRRHOSIS

The present prevailing view is that alcoholic cirrhosis develops in response to alcoholic hepatitis. As discussed before, the latter is characterized by ballooning of the hepatocytes, extensive necrosis, and polymorphonuclear inflammation. In addition, there is increased deposition of collagen and glycosaminoglycans (78). It is understandable that necrosis and inflammation may trigger the scarring process of cirrhosis, but one must question whether this is the only mechanism involved. In some populations, particularly in Europe and Japan (79,80), cirrhosis commonly develops in alcoholics without an apparent intermediate stage of florid alcoholic hepatitis. This observation raises the question whether alcohol can promote the development of cirrhosis without being preceded by alcoholic hepatitis. Indeed, in baboons fed alcohol, fatty liver developed, the hepatocytes increased in size, and there was some obvious ballooning. This ballooning was associated with some mononuclear inflammation but very few of the polymorphonuclear cells so characteristic of human alcoholic hepatitis (81). Although some clumping was apparent in the cytoplasm, by electron microscopy there was no alcoholic hyaline. Thus there was no florid picture of alcoholic hepatitis; yet, in one-third of the animals, typical cirrhosis developed (Figure 9). If one can extrapolate from these baboons to humans, it appears that full-blown alcoholic hepatitis may not be a necessary intermediate step in the

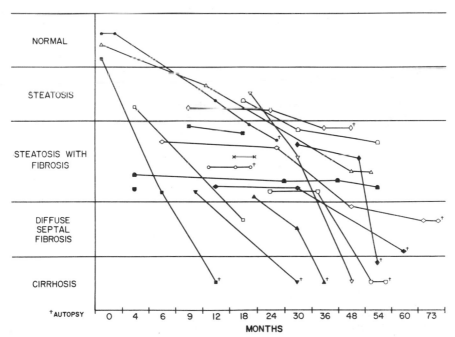

Figure 9. Sequential development of alcoholic liver injury. The most severe lesion is recorded individually for each time period in 18 baboons fed alcohol up to six years (1).

development of alcoholic cirrhosis. Preliminary sequential clinical observations support this contention.

This hypothesis in turn raises the question of which process, in the absence of alcoholic hepatitis, may initiate cirrhosis upon chronic consumption of ethanol. It is possible that cirrhosis develops in the presence of minimal inflammation and necrosis, which may suffice to trigger the fibrosis (82). On the other hand, it is also possible that, independent of the necrosis and inflammation, alcohol may have some more direct effects on the metabolism of collagen, the characteristic protein of the fibrous tissues.

In alcoholic liver injury there is a great variability in the magnitude of collagen deposition. At the earlier stages, in the so-called simple or uncomplicated fatty liver, collagen is detectable by chemical means only (83,84). When collagen deposition is sufficient to become visible by light microscopy, usually it appears first around the central (also called terminal) venules, resulting in so-called "pericentral" or "perivenular" fibrosis or sclerosis which extends into the lobule (perisinusoidal fibrosis). In cases of alcoholic hepatitis, Kent et al. (85) previously described an increased number of Ito cells. We now have recognized that even in the absence of alcoholic hepatitis, and prior to any fibrosis, some animals show an increased number of mesenchymal cells. Sequential biopsies in alcohol-fed baboons revealed that in some animals already at the early fatty liver stage an increased number of myofibroblasts and fibroblasts appear in the perivenular central areas (86). Myofibroblasts were found to be present in normal livers, but after ethanol, they proliferate in association with an increase in fibroblasts. This is eventually accompanied by deposition of abundant collagen bundles, first in the perivenular areas, leading to perivenular and pericellular fibrosis and ultimately to diffuse fibrosis and cirrhosis. Histochemically, procollagens and collagens type I and III are deposited with elastin and fibronectin; septa were accompanied by increases in laminin and collagen type IV (87). The myofibroblasts appear to play a key role in the overabundant deposition of collagen. They represent by far the most abundant mesenchymal cell in the perivenular area (86), and the composition of the fibrotic tissue suggests participation of a fibroblastic cell of wide biosynthetic potential, distinct from fibroblasts which usually do not synthesize basement membrane proteins. Myofibroblasts have been described in the fibrous tissue of human alcoholic cirrhosis (88) and, as mentioned before, myofibroblasts were also observed to increase in number in the alcohol-fed baboons in association with the development of fibrosis. Recent studies have revealed close similarities of the major structural components and their distribution in human (89) and baboon (87) alcoholic fibrosis.

In the experimental model of alcoholic liver injury in the baboon, an increased number of lipogranulomas was also found in the early stages (81). In man, too, some forms of lipogranulomas have been incriminated in the development of fibrosis (90). Thus, nonparenchymal (and perhaps parenchymal) cells participate in the production of collagen already at the fatty liver stage, but we do not know the respective role of parenchymal and nonparenchymal cells in this process.

The accumulation of hepatic collagen during the development of cirrhosis could theoretically be accomplished by increased synthesis, decreased degradation, or both.

Chronic ethanol consumption with adequate diets led to accumulation of hepatic collagen in rats and baboons, even when fibrosis was not yet histologically detectable (83). In the latter model, the role of increased collagen synthesis is suggested by increased activity of hepatic peptidylproline hydroxylase in rats and primates and increased incorporation of proline ^{14}C into hepatic collagen in rat liver slices (83). Increased hepatic peptidylproline hydroxylase activity was also found in patients with alcoholic cirrhosis (91), hepatitis (92), or in all stages of alcoholic liver disease (93). The role of increased collagen synthesis has been confirmed indirectly in man by autoradiographic techniques utilizing liver biopsies (94). A possible mechanism whereby alcohol consumption may be linked to collagen formation is the increase in tissue lactate secondary to alcohol metabolism (95) (Figure 5). Elevated concentrations of lactate have been associated with increased peptidylproline hydroxylase activity both in vitro (96) and in vivo (97). The hepatic free proline and pool size, which has been incriminated in the regulation of collagen synthesis (98,99), may be increased by ethanol (100) and is expanded in human portal cirrhosis (101). In patients with alcoholic cirrhosis, increased serum-free proline and hydroxyproline have been reported (102). Recently, it has again been postulated that lactate may play a role (103), this time through inhibition of proline oxidase (104). This hypothesis illustrates once more the possible impact of ethanol-induced redox changes on intermediary metabolism, including the metabolism of collagen.

SUMMARY

There are several main mechanisms that allow us to understand a number of the hepatic and metabolic effects of ethanol. Ethanol is oxidized in the liver to two products (hydrogen and acetaldehyde), to which many of the effects of ethanol can be attributed. The hydrogen generated alters the redox state, and though this effect is attenuated after chronic ethanol consumption, it may still be sufficient to explain alterations in lipid metabolism, possibly increased collagen deposition, and, under special circumstances, depression of protein synthesis. Acetaldehyde impairs microtubules, decreases protein secretion, and causes protein retention and ballooning of the hepatocyte. Acetaldehyde exerts toxicity also with regard to other key cellular functions, particularly in the mitochondria, and it may promote peroxidation of the cellular membranes. It is noteworthy that after chronic consumption of ethanol, there is increased acetaldehyde, in part because of decreased disposition in the mitochondria and partly because of induction of an alternative pathway of ethanol metabolism, namely the microsomal ethanol-oxidizing system. Indeed, this MEOS increases in activity after chronic ethanol consumption, with cross induction and acceleration of the metabolism of other drugs and increased lipoprotein production with hyperlipemia. There is also increased microsomal activation of hepatotoxic compounds (including drugs and possibly vitamin A). Fibrosis and cirrhosis can develop despite an associated adequate diet and even in the absence of alcoholic hepatitis. They are preceded by myofibroblasts and fibroblast proliferation. What eventually causes the increased number of myofibroblasts and promotes fibrosis is unclear, nor do we know the relative role of hepatocytes or mesenchymal cells in the process of fibroplasis. Possibly selective roles in this process of specific nutritional factors remain to be elucidated.

REFERENCES

1. C. S. Lieber, *Medical Disorders of Alcoholism: Pathogenesis and Treatment*, Saunders, Philadelphia, Pa., 1982, in press.
2. C. H. Best, W. S. Hartroft, C. S. Lucas, and J. H. Ridout, *Br. Med. J.*, **II,** 1001 (1949).
3. C. S. Lieber, D. P. Jones, and L. M. DeCarli, *J. Clin. Invest.*, **44,** 1009 (1965).
4. C. S. Lieber, D. P. Jones, J. Mendelson, and L. M. DeCarli, *Trans. Assoc. Am. Physicians*, **76,** 289 (1963).
5. L. M. DeCarli and C. S. Lieber, *J. Nutr.*, **91,** 331 (1967).
6. C. S. Lieber and L. M. DeCarli, *Am. J. Clin. Nutr.*, **23,** 474 (1970).
7. C. S. Lieber, L. M. DeCarli, H. Gang, G. Walker, and E. Rubin, in E. I. Goldsmith and J. Moor-Jankowski, Eds., *Medical Primatology*, part III, Karger, Basel, 1972, p. 270.
8. H. Popper and C. S. Lieber, *Am. J. Pathol.*, **98,** 695 (1980).
9. M. P. Salaspuro, W. A. Ross, E. Jayatilleke, S. Shaw and C. S. Lieber, *Hepatology*, **1,** 33 (1981).

10. C. S. Lieber and E. Rubin, *Am. J. Med.*, **44**, 200 (1968).

11. A. Iwamoto, E. E. Hellerstein, and D. M. Hegsted, *J. Nutr.*, **79**, 488 (1963).

12. C. S. Lieber and N. Spritz, *J. Clin. Invest.*, **45**, 1400 (1966).

13. C. S. Lieber and L. M. DeCarli, *Gastroenterology*, **50**, 316 (1966).

14. C. S. Lieber, A. Lefevre, N. Spritz, L. Feinman, and L. M. DeCarli, *J. Clin. Invest.*, **46**, 1451 (1967).

15. F. W. Hoffbauer and F. G. Zaki, *Acta. Pathol.*, **79**, 364 (1965).

16. W. Volwiler, C. M. Jones, and T. B. Mallory, *Gastroenterology*, **11**, 164 (1948).

17. J. Post, J. G. Benton, R. Breakstone, and J. Hoffman, *Gastroenterology*, **20**, 403 (1952)

18. G. B. Phillips and C. S. Davidson, *Ann. N.Y. Acad. Sci.*, **57**, 812 (1954).

19. R. E. Olson, in M. G. Wohl and R. S. Goodhart, Eds., *Modern Nutrition in Health and Disease*, Lea and Febiger, Philadelphia, 1964, p. 1037.

20. E. Rubin and C. S. Lieber, *New Engl. J. Med.*, **278**, 869 (1968).

21. N. R. Di Luzio, *Am. J. Phys.*, **194**, 453 (1958).

22. C. S. Lieber, *Fed. Proc.*, **26**, 1443 (1967).

23. G. Klatskin, W. A. Krehl, and H. O. Conn, *J. Exper. Med.*, **100**, 605 (1954).

24. C. S. Lieber, E. Rubin, and L. M. DeCarli, in V. M. Sardesai, Ed., *Biochemical and Clinical Aspects of Alcohol Metabolism*, C. C. Thomas, Springfield, Ill., 1969, p. 176.

25. C. S. Lieber, in E. E. Bittar, Ed., *The Biological Basis of Medicine*, Vol. 5, Chap. 4, Academic Press, New York, 1969, p. 317.

26. C. S. Lieber, N. Spritz, and L. M. DeCarli, *J. Clin. Invest.*, **45**, 51 (1966).

27. C. S. Lieber, N. Spritz, and L. M. DeCarli, *J. Lipid Res.*, **10**, 283 (1969).

28. K. N. Jeejeebhoy, A. Bruce-Robertson, J. Ho, and U. Sodtke, in M. A. Rothschild, M. Oratz, and S. S. Schreiber, Eds., *Alcohol and Abnormal Protein Synthesis*, Pergamon, New York, 1975, p. 373.

29. M. A. Rothschild, M. Oratz, J. Mongelli, and S. S. Schreiber, *J. Clin. Invest.*, **50**, 1812 (1971).

30. E. Baraona, P. Pikkarainen, M. Salaspuro, F. Finkelman, and C. S. Lieber, *Gastroenterology*, **79**, 104 (1980).

31. P. Jauhonen, E. Baraona, and C. S. Lieber, *Hepatology*, **1**, 520 (1981).

32. O. A. Iseri, C. S. Lieber, and L. S. Gottlieb, *Am. J. Pathol.*, **48**, 535 (1966).

33. B. P. Lane and C. S. Lieber, *Am. J. Pathol.*, **49**, 593 (1966).

34. E. Baraona, R. C. Pirola, and C. S. Lieber, *J. Clin. Invest.*, **52**, 296, (1973).

35. Y. Hasumura, R. Teschke, and C. S. Lieber, *Gastroenterology*, **66**, 415, (1974).

36. C. Sato, Y. Matsuda, and C. S. Lieber, *Gastroenterology*, **80**, 140 (1981).

37. M. A. Leo, M. Sato, and C. S. Lieber, *Clin. Res.*, **29**, 266 (1981).

38. M. Sato and C. S. Lieber, *J. Nutr.*, **111**, 2015 (1981).

39. M. A. Leo, M. Arai, M. Sato, and C. S. Lieber, *Gastroenterology*, **82**, 194 (1982).

40. C. S. Lieber, in M. Winick, Ed., *Nutrition and Gastroenterology*, Vol. 10, Wiley, New York, 1980, p. 153.

41. F. Nomura and C. S. Lieber, *Biochem. Biophys. Res. Commun.*, **100**, 131 (1981).

42. M. A. Korsten, S. Matsuzaki, L. Feinman, and C. S. Lieber, *New Engl. J. Med.*, **292**, 386 (1975).

43. K. O. Lindros, A. Stowell, P. Pikkarainen, and M. Salaspuro, *Pharm. Biochem. Behav.*, **13**, 119 (1980).

44. P. H. Pikkarainen, M. P. Salaspuro, and C. S. Lieber, *Alcoholism*, **3**, 259 (1979).

45. Y. Hasumura, R. Teschke and C. S. Lieber, *J. Biol. Chem.*, **251** 4908 (1976).

46. E. Rubin and C. S. Lieber, *Gastroenterology*, **52**, 1 (1967).

47. O. R. Koch, A. Boveris, S. Sirotzky De Favelukes, M. Schwarcz de Tarlovsky, and A. O. M. Stoppani, *Exper. Molec. Pathol.*, **27**, 213 (1977).

48. E. Rubin, D. S. Beattie, and C. S. Lieber, *Lab. Invest.*, **23**, 620 (1970).

49. M. C. Oudea, A. N. Launay, S. Queneherve, and P. Oudea, *Rev. Eur. Etudes Clin. Biol.*, **15**, 748 (1970).

50. E. R. Gordon, *J. Biol. Chem.*, **248**, 8271 (1973).

51. Y. Hasumura, R. Teschke, and C. S. Lieber, *Science*, **189**, 727 (1975).

52. K. H. Kiessling and L. Pilstrom, *Quart. J. Stud. Alcohol*, **29**, 819 (1968).

53. E. Rubin, D. S. Beattie, A. Toth, and C. S. Lieber, *Fed. Proc.*, **31**, 131 (1972).

54. E. A. Hosein, I. Hofmann, and E. Linder, *Arch. Biochem. Biophys.*, **183** (1977).

55. S. Wahid, J. M. Khanna, F. J. Carmichael, and Y. Israel, *Res. Commun. Chem. Path. Pharmacol.*, **30**, 477 (1980).

56. A. I. Cederbaum, C. S. Lieber, and E. Rubin, *Biochem. Biophys.*, **165**, 560 (1974).

57. A. I. Cederbaum, C. S. Lieber, and E. Rubin, *Arch. Biochem. Biophys.*, **161**, 26 (1974).

58. H. Sprince, C. M. Parker, G. Smith, and L. J. Gonzales, *Agents and Actions*, **4**, 125 (1974).

59. A. I. Cederbaum and E. Rubin, *Biochem. Pharmacol.*, **25**, 963 (1976).

60. S. Shaw, E. Jayatilleke, W. A. Ross, E. R. Gordon, and C. S. Lieber, *J. Lab. Clin. Med.*, **98**, 417 (1981).

61. A. Wendel, S. Fenerstein, and K. H. Konz, *Biochem. Phys.*, **28**, 2051 (1979).

62. N. R. DiLuzio and T. E. Stege, in M. M. Fisher and J. G. Rankin, Eds., *Alcohol and the Liver*, Vol. 3, Plenum, New York, 1977, p. 45.

63. N. R. DiLuzio and A. D. Hartman, *Fed. Proc.*, **26**, 1436 (1967).

64. J. Bunyan, M. A. Cawthrone, A. T. Diplock, and J. Green, *Br. J. Nutr.*, **23**, 309 (1969).

65. M. Comporti, E. Burdino, and F. Raja, *Life Sci.*, **10** (Part II), 855 (1971).

66. S. Hashimoto and R. O. Recknagel, *Exp. Mol. Pathol.*, **8**, 225 (1968).

67. R. Scheig and G. Klatskin, *Life Sci.*, **8**, 855 (1969).

68. C. S. Lieber and L. M. DeCarli, *Science*, **170**, 78 (1970).

69. R. C. Reitz, *Biochem. Biophys. Acta*, **380**, 145 (1975).

70. C. M. MacDonald, *FEBS Lett.*, **35**, 227 (1973).

71. C.-P. Sieger, A. Schütt, and O. Strubelt, *Proc. Eur. Soc. Toxicol.*, **18**, 160 (1977).

72. C. S. Lieber, D. P. Jones, and L. M. DeCarli, *J. Clin. Invest.*, **44**, 1009 (1965).

73. E. Baraona, M. A. Leo, S. A. Borowsky, and C. S. Lieber, *Science*, **190**, 794 (1975).

74. Y. Matsuda, E. Baraona, M. Salaspuro, and C. S. Lieber, *Lab. Invest.*, **41**, 455 (1979).

75. D. H. Gregory, Z. R. Vlahcevic, M. F. Prugh, and L. Swell, *Gastroenterology*, **74**, 93 (1978).

76. E. Baraona, M. A. Leo, S. A. Borowsky, and C. S. Lieber, *J. Clin. Invest.*, **50**, 546 (1977).

77. H. Orrego, L. M. Blendis, I. R. Crossley, A. Medline, A. MacDonald, S. Ritchie, and Y. Israel, *Gastroenterology*, **80**, 546 (1981).

78. J. T. Galambos and R. Shapiro, *J. Clin. Invest.*, **52**, 2952 (1973).

79. E. Inoue, *Gastroenterol. Japonica*, **12**, 230 (1966).

80. M. Sakurai, *Acta Pathol. Jpn.*, **19**, 283 (1969).

81. H. Popper and C. S. Lieber, *Am. J. Pathol.*, **98**, 695 (1980).

82. C. S. Lieber, in M. M. Fisher and J. G. Rankin, Eds., *Pathogenesis of Alcoholic Liver Disease: An Overview*, Vol. 3, Plenum, New York, 1977, p. 197.

83. L. Feinman and C. S. Lieber, *Science*, **176**, 795 (1972).

84. A. J. Patek, S. C. Bowry, and S. M. Sabesin, *Arch. Pathol. Lab. Med.*, **100**, 19 (1976).

85. G. Kent, S. Gay, T. Inouye, R. Bahu, O. T. Minick, and H. Popper, *Proc. Nat. Acad. Sci. USA*, **73**, 3719 (1976).

86. M. Nakano and C. S. Lieber, *Am. J. Pathol.*, **106**, 145 (1982).

87. E. G. Hahn, R. Timpl, M. Nakano, and C. S. Lieber, *Gastroenterology*, **79**, 1025 (1980).

88. P. S. Bhathal, *Pathology*, **4**, 139 (1972).

89. E. G. Hahn, G. Wick, D. Pencev, and R. Timpl, *Gut*, **21**, 63 (1980).

90. P. Christoffersen, O. Brendstrup, E. Juhl, and H. Poulsen, *Acta Path. Microbiol. Scand.*, **79**, 150 (1971).

91. R. S. Patrick, *J. Alcoholism*, **8**, 13 (1973)

92. E. Mezey, J. J. Potter, F. L. Iber, and W. C. Maddrey, *J. Lab. Clin. Med.*, **93**, 92 (1979).

93. S. W. Mann, G. C. Fuller, J. V. Rodil, and E. I. Vidins, *Gut*, **20**, 825 (1979).

94. T. S. N. Chen and C. M. Leevy, *J. Lab. Clin. Med.*, **85**, 103 (1975).

95. C. S. Lieber, E. Rubin, and L. M. DeCarli, in B. Kissin and H. Begleiter, Eds., *The Biology of Alcoholism*, Vol. 1, Plenum, New York, 1971, p. 263.

96. H. Green and B. Goldberg, *Nature*, **204**, 347 (1964).

97. S. Lindy, F. B. Pedersen, H. Turto, and J. Uitto, *Hoppe-Seylers' Z. Physiol. Chem.*, **352**, 1113 (1971).

98. M. Chvapil and J. N. Ryan, *Agents and Actions*, **3**, 38 (1973).

99. M. Rojkind, M. and L. Diaz De Leon, *Biochem. Biophys. Acta*, **217**, 512 (1970).

100. H.-M. Hakkinen and E. Kulonen, *Biochem. Pharmacol.*, **24**, 199 (1975).

101. D. Kershenobich, F. J. Fierro, and M. Rojkind, *J. Clin. Invest.*, **49**, 2246 (1970).

102. J. M. Mata, D. Kershenobich, E. Villarreal, and M. Rojkind, *Gastroenterology*, **68**, 1265 (1975).

103. D. Kershenobich, G. Garcia-Tsao, S. A. Saldana, and M. Rojkind, *Gastroenterology*, **80**, 1012 (1981).

104. E. M. Kowaloff, J. M. Phang, A. S. Granger, and S. J. Downing, *Proc. Natl. Acad. Sci. U.S.A.*, **74**, 5368 (1971).

105. C. S. Lieber, *Pharmacol. Biochem. Behav.*, **13**, 17 (1980).

5

Drugs and Vitamin B_{12} and Folate Metabolism

JOHN LINDENBAUM, M.D.

Harlem Hospital Center, Columbia University, College of Physicians and Surgeons, New York, New York

It is appropriate that the effects of drugs on the metabolism of folate (folic acid) and on that of cobalamin (vitamin B_{12}) be discussed together because of the many associations between the two vitamins. Deficiency of either interferes with DNA synthesis and may result in megaloblastic anemia, thrombocytopenia, leukopenia, atrophic glossitis, and megaloblastic changes in other organs that have rapid cell turnover and continuing requirements for DNA synthesis, such as the gastrointestinal tract or the uterine cervix. Treatment with one vitamin may ameliorate these signs of deficiency even when they are due to lack of the other. But there are many ways in which they differ. Not only do the two vitamins have rather dissimilar molecular structures, but they are present in different foods, absorbed at different sites in the gastrointestinal tract, utilize different transport systems, and are metabolized and excreted at different rates (1,2). Most intriguing, perhaps, is the central and peripheral nervous system demyelinating disorder that appears to be exclusive to cobalamin deficiency, despite continuing anecdotal reports of neuropathy attributed to folate deficiency. In the following discussion *metabolism* will be interpreted broadly to include the absorption, biochemical transformations, utilization, and excretion of the vitamins, and *drugs* to denote not only compounds marketed by pharmaceutical companies, but other foreign agents, such as ethanol and general anesthetics. A distinction will be made between interactions in which the administration of a drug actually contributes to the development of a deficiency state that results in an illness, and those interactions which are of no clinical importance. It will be apparent that virtually all the clinically important drug–vitamin interactions involve folic acid rather than cobalamin.

73

Table 1.   Causes of Folate Deficiency in 201 Consecutive Cases of Megaloblastic Anemia in New York City[a]

Cause	Number of Cases
Alcoholism and poor diet[b]	180 (89.6%)
Poor diet	4 (2.0%)
Sprue syndromes	13 (6.4%)
Pregnancy (nonalcoholic)	2 (1.0%)
Sulfasalazine	1 (0.5%)
? Oral contraceptives	1 (0.5%)

[a]Patients admitted to Harlem or Presbyterian Hospitals, 1968–1978 (3).
[b]Includes three pregnant patients, four patients taking phenytoin, and two patients with cancer.

DRUG–FOLATE INTERACTIONS

In a recent consecutive series (3) of patients with anemia associated with a megaloblastic bone marrow, low serum folate concentrations, and a subsequent response to folic acid therapy (Table 1), the combination of alcohol ingestion and poor dietary folate intake was responsible for approximately 90% of cases. In a small number of patients, the administration of phenytoin or sulphasalazine may have contributed to the development of folate deficiency. Patients with megalobalstic change due to treatment of malignancies with methotrexate were excluded from this series. With this proviso, the interaction between ethanol and folate was clearly the most important cause of deficiency of the vitamin, and will therefore be discussed first.

Alcohol

The association between chronic alcohol intake and folic acid deficiency has long been recognized, and is the subject of several recent reviews (4–6). The incidence of megaloblastic anemia in various published series of alcoholic patients varies from less than 1% to 40%, depending on patient selection. The most important factor favoring the appearance of significant folate deficiency is poor dietary intake of the vitamin (4,6). Clinically important lack of folate is only very rarely seen in well-nourished alcoholics. Megaloblastic anemia in alcoholics is always due to folate deficiency, unless some other underlying condition resulting in cobalamin depletion (such as pernicious anemia) is present. The presence of megaloblastic anemia does not correlate well with the severity of alcohol-associated hepatic dysfunction. It is more common in wine and whiskey drinkers than in imbibers of beer, which is rich in the vitamin (again suggesting the importance of dietary folate intake in the pathogenesis of this complication). The diagnostic problems associated with megaloblastic anemia in alcoholics, including the tendency of megaloblastic changes in the neutrophil series to persist in the bone marrow and peripheral blood after the erythroid marrow has become normoblastic, are discussed elsewhere (3,4).

In addition, many alcoholics have low serum folate levels (and in some cases low erythrocyte concentrations of the vitamin) in the absence of morphologic evidence of depletion of tissue stores. Serum folate tends to be inversely related to serum ethanol concentrations (7).

The cause of the high incidence of folate deficiency in alcoholics is not poor diet alone. Sullivan and Herbert clearly demonstrated that alcohol acts as a weak folate antagonist (8). The administration of ethanol along with small doses of folic acid to patients recovering from megabloblastic anemia prevented the hematologic response to folic acid therapy. The heamtosuppressive effect could be overcome with larger doses of folic or folinic acid (8). Subsequently, other investigators were also able to induce megaloblastic marrow abnormalities by the administration of ethanol and folate-poor diet to human volunteers (1). These morphologic changes do not occur when alcohol is given with folate supplements to well-nourished volunteers (9,10). Eichner and Hillman also found that when alcohol was given along with a low-folate diet, megaloblastic marrow conversion occurred much more rapidly than when the diet alone was taken (11).

There is some evidence that malabsorption of folic acid may play a role in the development of folate deficiency (5,12). Alcohol intoxication and folate deficiency appear to act synergistically to depress small bowel function (5). Romero and co-workers have recently reported that chronic ethanol feeding to monkeys along with folic acid supplements results in malabsorption of folic acid (13). However alcohol administration in humans does not depress the intestinal absorption of folic acid unless a folate-poor diet is given simultaneously (4,5). The evidence suggests that folate malabsorption in alcoholic patients is the result of small bowel dysfunction due to folate deficiency itself (6).

In an important study, Eichner and Hillman observed that the acute intravenous administration of ethanol to fasting, well-nourished human volunteers caused a rapid fall in serum folate concentrations within six hours (14). In rats, bile drainage also causes an acute fall in serum folate (15). Hillman and co-workers hypothesized that alcohol lowers serum folate concentrations by interrupting the enterohepatic cycle of the vitamin. They presented evidence that when ethanol was given for three days to rats deprived of folate, the clearance of intravenously administered radiolabeled folic acid into bile was decreased, with retention of the label in the liver and increased formation of hepatic polyglutamate folates (16). Other investigators, however, using different experimental conditions (Table 2), have reported conflicting results (17,18). The relevance of any of these studies to the situation in acute and chronic alcoholism in humans is uncertain. In isolated rat hepatocytes, ethanol was recently shown to cause an increased uptake of 5-methyltetrahydrofolate, the main form of folate present in human serum (19). It is likely that alcohol interferes in some way with the hepatic processing and/or enterohepatic circulation of folate, but the exact locus and nature of the lesion remains to be established.

Whatever the mechanism, it has been shown that when the inexpensive wines most commonly ingested by alcoholics who develop deficiency are fortified by the inclusion of folic acid, the added folate is well absorbed, even by intoxicated patients, and this has been proposed as a simple and cheap way of preventing the morbidity and mortality of megaloblastic anemia in alcoholics (20).

Alcohol intoxication is associated with a number of other hematologic complications. Sideroblastic changes in the bone marrow are almost as common as megaloblastic hematopoiesis, and the two are frequently found in the same patient (3,7,21). It has been argued that folate deficiency is a necessary precondition for the development of ring

Table 2. Effect of Ethanol Feeding on Hepatic Folate Metabolism After Injection of 3H-PGA

Reference	Animal	Duration of Alcohol Feeding	Pentaglutamate Synthesis	Hepatic Retention of Label
Brown et al. (17)	Rat	14 days	Decreased	Decreased
Hillman et al. (16)	Folate-deprived Rat			
Tamura et al. (18)	Monkey	1-2 years	Normal	Decreased

sideroblasts in the bone marrow in such patients (22), but in some, sideroblastic anemia appears to develop in the absence of evidence of concomitant lack of folate (3). Alcohol intoxication is also very commonly associated with a macrocytosis that is *not* accompanied by evidence of folate deficiency. The cause of this complication is not established (4). Thrombocytopenia, vacuolization of marrow precursor cells, neutropenia, and impairment of granulocyte mobilization may also occur after ethanol intoxication in the absence of coexisting folate deficiency (6).

Sulfasalazine

Megaloblastic anemia due to folate deficiency has occasionally been reported in patients with inflammatory bowel disease (ulcerative colitis and regional enteritis), and has been attributed to various mechanisms, including poor dietary intake, impaired absorption, and (possibly) increased tissue utilization of folate (23). Low serum and/or red cell folate levels have also been found in a variable percentage of patients with inflammatory bowel disorders (23,24). Sulfasalazine, a compound containing a sulfa drug and a salicylate that is broken down to its active components by the gut flora, is widely used in the treatment of inflammatory bowel disease, and has been shown to impair the absorption of folic acid (23,25), polyglutamyl folate (25), and methyl-tetrahydrofolic acid (24) in patients with these disorders. The drug was also found to interfere with the absorption of orally administered pteroyglutamic acid in normal volunteers (23). The effect on folate absorption, although definite, was variable and often only slight to moderate in degree (23,24). In several recent case reports (24,26,27), megaloblastic anemia has been attributed at least in part to the action of the drug on folate absorption, although it has been argued that since the effects of the agent on folate absorption are usually not profound, it will play a contributory role only in patients in whom other factors causing folate deficiency, such as poor diet or upper intestinal disease, are present (24). However, we have encountered two patients within the last three years with inflammatory bowel disease without evidence of poor diet or upper intestinal involvement who have developed a mild macrocytic anemia associated with low serum folate concentrations while on sulfasalazine. In each case the anemia and macrocytosis responded to folic acid therapy while the drug was continued. Sulfasalazine therapy may also cause a mild hemolytic state, which may contribute to macrocytosis by increasing the number of immature circulating erythrocytes (24,28), and conceivably may increase folate requirements (28).

The drug inhibits the uptake of monoglutamate and polyglutamate folates by the small bowel (23,25). The effect on monoglutamate uptake can be shown by using everted rings of rat jejunum in vitro, and appears to be due to the intact compound rather than its active metabolites (23). Similarly, the intact molecule, but not its component parts, has been shown to inhibit the human brush border enzyme, folate conjugase, that hydrolyzes polyglutamate folates (29). The drug also weakly inhibits a number of enzymes which catalyze reactions requiring different folate coenzymes, suggesting that it interferes with a common folate recognition site (30,31). Whether this action could contribute to the development of megaloblastic anemia (in addition to the effect on intestinal transport) is uncertain.

Anticonvulsants

There is considerable evidence suggesting an interaction between anticonvulsant drugs and folate balance, although the nature of the disturbance has not yet been elucidated and it is rarely of clinical importance. In many published series, a substantial percentage of patients receiving anticonvulsant therapy for epilepsy have subnormal serum, red cell, and cerebrospinal fluid folate levels (1). In addition, macrocytosis (unassociated with anemia) is extremely common in such patients (1). On the other hand, clinically significant folate deficiency (i.e., megaloblastic anemia) is rare, occurring in less than 1% of patients taking these drugs. Most of the reported patients have received phenytoin, but the complication has been seen with several other anticonvulsants, including phenobarbital and primidone. In the patients with megaloblastic anemia, other factors promoting the development of folate deficiency, such as poor diet and alcoholism, have often been present. The only patients we have seen over the past decade in New York City with folate-deficiency megaloblastic anemia associated with such drugs were four alcoholics who were eating poorly as well as taking phenytoin (Table 1).

The mechanism of the interaction between folate and anticonvulsants has been the subject of many studies, but is poorly understood. Early claims that phenytoin interfered with the absorption of polyglutamate forms of folate (32–34) have not been substantiated by others (35–37). Several laboratories have reported impairment of the absorption of folic acid in monoglutamate form and an equal number have demonstrated no effect (31,38–41). Virtually all of the conflicting reports have used different methods of studying folate absorption, yielding results that are not entirely comparable. It is likely that there is no effect of phenytoin on monoglutamate absorption, or that is produces only a mild interference with intestinal uptake. A slight effect would be consistent with the observation that most patients show subclinical evidence of deficiency and that only a rare patient, usually with other contributing disorders, develops full-blown megaloblastic anemia.

It is also possible that anticonvulsant therapy affects folate metabolism. The administration of phenytoin (but not phenobarbitone) to mice increased the urinary excretion of folate catabolites from the second, or late-appearing, folate metabolic pool (42). In contrast, in a single human volunteer studied by a different method, phenytoin appeared to accelerate the rate of folate elimination from the early, or short-lived, pool without affecting the second pool (43).

Folic acid therapy may cause a variable depression in serum phenytoin concentrations (31,44). Striking individual case reports have appeared in which folic acid administration appeared to precipitate seizures in epileptic patients receiving anticonvulsants. However, many well-controlled trials have shown no effect of supplemental folic acid therapy on the frequency of fits (45). Very large doses of folic acid in the absence of anticonvulsant therapy may cause seizures, especially if injected into the central nervous system (46); similar effects have been reported with other folate derivatives, including folate antagonists, and the relevance to humans of studies showing an interaction between phenytoin and various forms of folate in the production of seizures in rats (16) is uncertain.

It is of interest that not all patients who develop macrocytosis while on anticonvulsant drugs have subnormal serum and red cell folate levels or biochemical evidence of folate deficiency when bone marrow DNA synthesis is studied in vitro (47). The situation thus parallels that seen with alcohol, which may cause macrocytosis that is related or apparently unrelated to folate deficiency (4); this may also occur with sulfasalazine (24,28).

Dihydrofolate Reductase Inhibitors

Methotrexate, a drug extensively used in the treatment of cancer and severe psoriasis, is a very effective inhibitor of dihydrofolate reductase, the enzyme which catalyzes the conversion of dihydrofolate to tetrahydrofolate, as well as that of folic acid to dihydrofolate (Figure 1).

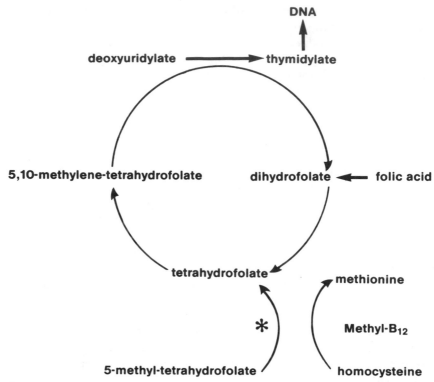

Figure 1.   The de novo synthesis of thymidylate (upper part of figure) requires a folate coenzyme, 5, 10-methylene-tetrahydrofolate. The dihydrofolate reductase inhibitor drugs decrease the supply of this cofactor by inhibiting the conversion of folic acid to dihydrofolate and the subsequent reduction of dihydrofolate to tetrahydrofolate. The methionine synthetase reaction (asterisk) requires methylcobalamin as a cofactor. If this step is blocked, as in vitamin B$_{12}$ deficiency or after prolonged nitrous oxide anesthesia, the supply of tetrahydrofolate will be reduced and cellular folate will be "trapped" in the form of 5-methyl-tetrahydrofolate.

Although this is its primary locus of action in interfering with DNA synthesis, there are a number of secondary effects on cellular metabolism, such as inhibition of thymidylate synthetase and depletion of cellular folates (48–50). Detailed discussion of this group of agents is beyond the scope of this chapter. Note, however, that a number of other drugs used for other purposes are weak inhibitors of dihydrofolate reductase, or have a much stronger affinity for bacterial or protozoal than for human reductases. These compounds are listed in Table 3. Each of these agents has been shown to inhibit the human enzyme in vitro. Pyrimethamine,

Table 3.   Weak Inhibitors of Dihydrofolate
Reductase that Rarely Cause Megaloblastic
Anemia

Drug	Clinical Use
Pyrimethamine	Antimalarial
Pentamidine	Antiprotozoal
Trimethoprim	Antibacterial, antiprotozoal
Triamterene	Diuretic

pentamidine, trimethoprim, and (possibly) triamterene have all been shown occasionally to cause megaloblastic anemia in patients (48,51). This is particularly likely to be encountered at high dosage, and in patients with preexisting depletion of folate stores due to other underlying conditions, such as pregnancy, poor diet, or chronic alcoholism.

Oral Contraceptives

A number of cases of megaloblastic anemia due to folate deficiency have been reported in women taking oral contraceptive agents (52), although when one considers the large number of women taking these drugs, the incidence must be very low indeed. While in some cases no apparent cause for the megaloblastic anemia other than contraceptive therapy was demonstrated, in many patients other underlying disorders that were likely to disturb folate balance, such as celiac disease, decreased dietary vitamin intake, and the administration of other drugs known to affect folate status, have also been present (52). Thus it is uncertain whether these agents are truly associated with the risk of developing megaloblastic anemia. There are conflicting reports in the literature as to whether women on these agents have lowered serum or red cell folate levels (52,53). There is no convincing evidence that sex steroids affect folate absorption (52). About 20% of women taking contraceptive hormones were found to have mild megaloblastic changes on Papanicolaou smears of the cervicovaginal epithelium (in the absence of systemic folate deficiency) (52). These changes disappeared after folic acid therapy, suggesting that oral contraceptives may cause an increased demand for folate limited to the reproductive system (52). The changes have not yet been shown to have any clinical significance.

Cholestyramine

Long-term treatment with the nonabsorbable anion exchange resin cholestyramine, which has been used in the management of hypercholesterolemia, pruritis, and diarrhea following ileal resection, may be associated with low serum and red cell folate concentrations (54). Although an effect on folate absorption has not yet been shown experimentally, it is possible that this agent interferes with monoglutamate or polyglutamate absorption (or enterohepatic recycling) as a result of its ability to bind anions. It has not yet been shown to cause megaloblastic anemia.

DRUG–COBALAMIN INTERACTIONS

Cobalamins are extensively stored in the body and a period of several years of deprivation is typically required to produce a clinically significant deficiency state (1). Many drugs have been well shown to inhibit the absorption of vitamin B_{12} in humans (57–62) (Table 4). However, the development of megaloblastic anemia or neurological disorders secondary to cobalamin deficiency as a result of the administration of any of these medications does not seem to occur, or has been described only in rare case reports in which the documentation of the cause and effect relation of the drug to the deficiency state was problematic or incomplete (63,64). This appears to be the case because (1) each of these agents causes only a partial block in cobalamin absorption, and (2) many years of drug administration would be required to deplete body stores of the vitamin in a previously normal person. In addition, several of the drugs in question are not currently widely used, and (in the case of some of

Table 4.   Drugs that Impair Cobalamin Absorption

Drug	Reference Number
Biguanides	55,56,64
Cholestyramine	57
Colchicine	58
Ethanol	59
Neomycin	60
Para-aminosalicylic acid	61,63
Potassium chloride	62

them) larger than usual doses may need to be given in order to impair cobalamin absorption.

Vitamin C

Considerable contoversy has been generated by a report that high doses of vitamin C could destroy the vitamin B_{12} in homogenized meals when studied in vitro (64a). Evidence has been presented that destruction of food cobalamins by ascorbic acid can be shown only when vitamin B_{12} is assayed in the absence of cyanide extraction (65,66), and it has been argued that the effect is therefore merely an in vitro artifact (65). In vivo studies of the effect of ascorbic acid on the absorption of cobalamins in food will be required to resolve this controversy, which so far has generated more heat than light. Unequivocal cases of megaloblastic anemia due to ascorbic acid ingestion have not yet been reported, and it has not been shown in controlled studies that long-term ascorbate therapy reduces serum cobalamin levels (67).

Oral Contraceptives

Although it has not been a universal finding (52), a number of groups have reported low serum cobalamin levels, as measured microbiologically or by radioassay, in women using oral contraceptive agents (68,69). Even in the absence of subnormal values, the mean serum B_{12} concentration of women using these drugs may be lower than that of controls (68). Conflicting data have been reported concerning the effect of sex steroid therapy on serum cobalamin-binding proteins (52,68,69). None of the reported patients with low serum concentrations had any evidence of deficiency, and oral contraceptives do not impair the absorption of vitamin B_{12} (69). Thus the low cobalamin level occasionally seen in women on oral contraceptives appears to be a laboratory abnormality of uncertain cause and of no clinical significance.

Nitrous Oxide

A recently recognized interaction between nitrous oxide and vitamin B_{12} has been partly elucidated at the biochemical level and appears to have major implications for our understanding of the mechanism of action of cobalamins and the nature of folate–B_{12} interrelations. There have been two parallel but independent lines of clinical observation of the effects of nitrous oxide on cobalamin metabolism, one hematologic and the other neurologic. Twenty-five years ago Lassen and co-workers observed that patients receiving prolonged nitrous oxide anesthesia in the treatment of tetanus developed acute granulocytopenia, thrombocytopenia, and megaloblastic hematopoiesis in bone marrow aspirates (70). In patients receiving nitrous oxide daily for several weeks fatalities due to bone marrow failure were observed. These workers then undertook a trial of daily nitrous oxide therapy in the management of chronic myelogenous leukemia, which resulted in transient, incomplete remissions as well as unacceptable side effects (71). These observations evoked little interest until 1976 when Amess and co-workers "rediscovered" that nitrous oxide induced megaloblastic hematopoiesis in studies of patients receiving the anesthetic for 24 hours during cardiac bypass surgery (72). Studies of in vitro DNA synthesis by incubated bone marrow for such patients showed a pattern typical of vitamin B $_{12}$ deficiency (73). Rapid recovery of bone marrow morphology and function occurred after cessation of anesthesia, and there was no evidence of nervous system damage that could be attributed to impairment of cobalamin metabolism.

In contrast, there have been an increasing number of case reports of neurologic damage in the absence of any hematologic abnormalities in people who abuse nitrous oxide (74,75). The patient population involved have been dentists, anesthetists, or laymen who inhale the anesthetic for short periods of time in order to experience "highs" on a chronic, daily basis. After such prolonged, but less intensive exposure, serious neurologic disorders have occurred which in a number of instances have mimicked the findings seen in patients with pernicious anemia or other causes of long-standing cobalamin deficiency.

The cobalt atom in the center of the corrin ring of the vitamin B $_{12}$ coenzymes is most likely in a 2-electron reduced form (Co^+) that is oxidized to Co^{3+} by nitrous oxide. Exposure of animals to nitrous oxide results in an acute decrease in the activity of methionine synthetase (76,77), one of the two enzyme systems in mammalian systems known to require a cobalamin coenzyme (methyl-B $_{12}$). This is likely to be the result of displacement of methylcobalamin from methionine synthetase, presumably as a result of the oxidation of the cobalt atom (77).

The biochemical lesion thought to be the basis for the megaloblastic hematopoiesis seen in cobalamin deficiency (78) is shown in the lower part of Figure 1. The asterisk indicates the methionine synthetase reaction. Methyl-B $_{12}$ promotes the conversion of 5-methyl-tetrahydrofolate to tetrahydrofolate, which can then undergo further modifications, ultimately resulting in the conversion of deoxyuridylate to deoxythymidylate, which is incorporated into DNA. In the absence of cobalamin, the cell accumulates 5-methyl-tetrahydrofolate, a form of folate that cannot be used in DNA synthesis. Therefore the oxidation of the cobalt atom in methyl-B_{12} causes acute megaloblastic hematopoiesis.

What, then, is the explanation of the neurologic lesion seen in vitamin B_{12} deficiency or after chronic low-dose nitrous oxide exposure? Scott and co-workers have recently reported that chronic exposure of monkeys to nitrous oxide results in severe central nervous system damage that resembles that seen in subacute combined degeneration due to cobalamin deficiency (79). These neurological lesions were markedly ameliorated by the coadministration of methionine with the anesthetic (79). The findings suggest that the neuropathy of cobalamin deficiency is due to methionine deficiency secondary to inactivation of methionine synthetase. If this explanation is correct, it may explain why nervous system damage is seen in cobalamin deficiency states but not in those due to lack of folate, and why folic acid therapy improves hematopoiesis but usually does not ameliorate the nervous system damage in patients with vitamin B_{12} deficiency. There are still many unanswered questions (78), but the nitrous oxide cobalamin interaction has provided a convenient experimental model in which vitamin B_{12} deficiency can be induced acutely in animals, without requiring prolonged experiments to deplete body stores of the vitamin.

REFERENCES

1. I. Chanarin, *The Megaloblastic Anaemias*, Blackwell, Philadelphia, 1969.
2. J. Lindenbaum, in R. E. Hodges, Ed., *Nutrition: Metabolic and Clinical Applications*, Plenum, New York, pp. 1–51.
3. J. Lindenbaum and M. A. Roman, *Am. J. Clin. Nutr.*, **33**, 2727 (1980).
4. J. Lindenbaum, *Semin. Hematol.*, **17**, 119 (1980).
5. C. H. Halsted and T. Tamura, in C. S. Davidson, Ed., *Problems in Liver Diseases*, Stratton, New York, 1979, pp. 91–100.
6. J. Lindenbaum, Chapter 8, in C. S. Lieber, *Medical Disorders of Alcoholism*, Saunders, New York, 1982, in press.
7. E. R. Eichner, and R. S. Hillman, *Am. J. Med.*, **50**, 218 (1971).
8. L. W. Sullivan and V. Herbert, *J. Clin. Invest.*, **43**, 2048 (1964).
9. J. Lindenbaum and C. S. Lieber, *New Engl. J. Med.*, **281**, 333 (1969).
10. D. H. Cowan, *J. Lab. Clin Med.*, **81**, 64 (1973).
11. E. R. Eichner, H. I. Pierce and R. S. Hillman, *New Engl. J. Med.*, **284**, 933 (1971).
12. F. A. Klipstein and J. Lindenbaum, *Blood*, **25**, 443 (1965).
13. J. J. Romero, T. Tamura, and C. H. Halsted, *Gastroenterol.*, **80**, 99 (1981).

14. E. R. Eichner and R. S. Hillman, *J. Clin. Invest.*, **52,** 584 (1973).

15. S. E. Steinberg, C. L. Campbell, and R. S. Hillman, *J. Clin. Invest.*, **64,** 83 (1979).

16. R. S. Hillman, R. McGriffin, and C. Campbell, *Trans. Assoc. Amer. Phys.*, **90,** 145 (1977).

17. J. P. Brown, G. E. Davidson, and J. M. Scott, *Biochem. Pharmacol.*, **22,** 3287 (1973).

18. T. Tamura, J. J. Romero, J. E. Watson, E. J. Gong, and C. H. Halsted, *J. Lab. Clin. Med.*, **97,** 654 (1981).

19. D. W. Horne, W. T. Briggs, and C. Wagner, *Arch. Biochem. Biophys.*, **196,** 557 (1979).

20. J. D. Kaunitz and J. Lindenbaum, *Ann. Intern. Med.*, **87,** 542 (1977).

21. J. D. Hines, *Br. J. Haematol.*, **16,** 87 (1969).

22. H. I. Pierce, R. G. McGuffin, and R. S. Hillman, *Arch. Intern. Med.*, **136,** 283 (1976).

23. J. L. Franklin and I. H. Rosenberg, *Gastroenterology*, **64,** 517 (1973).

24. C. W. Swinson, J. Perry, M. Lumb, and A. J. Levi, *Gut*, **22,** 456 (1981).

25. C. H. Halsted, G. Gandhi, and T. Tamura, *New Engl. J. Med.*, *305*, 1513 (1981).

26. R. E. Schneider and L. Beeley, *Br. Med. J.*, **2,** 1638 (1977).

27. S. P. Kane and M. A. Boots, *Br. Med. J.*, **4,** 1287 (1977).

28. R. E. Pounder, E. R. Craven, J. S. Henthorn, and J. M. Bannayne, *Gut*, **16,** 181 (1975).

29. A. M. Reisenauer and C. H. Halsted, *Biochim. Biophys. Acta*, **659,** 62 (1981).

30. J. Selhub, G. J. Dhar, and I. H. Rosenberg, *J. Clin. Invest.*, **61,** 221 (1978).

31. C. L. Baum, J. Selhub, and I. H. Rosenberg, *J. Lab. Clin. Med.*, **97,** 779 (1981).

32. A. V. Hoffbrand and T. F. Necheles, *Lancet*, **2,** 528 (1968).

33. I. H. Rosenberg, H. A. Godwin, R. R. Streiff, and W. B. Castle, *Lancet*, **2,** 530 (1968).

34. P. Reizenstein and L. Lund, *Scand. J. Haemat.*, **11,** 158 (1973).

35. C. Fehling, M. Jagerstad, K. Lindstrand, and A. K. Westesson, *Clin. Sci.*, **44,** 595 (1973).

36. C. M. Houlihan, J. M. Scott, P. H. Boyle, and D. G. Weir, *Gut*, **13,** 189 (1972).

37. J. Perry and I. Chanarin, *Gut*, **13,** 544 (1972).

38. A. Benn, C. H. J. Swan, W. T. Cooke, J. A. Blair, A. J. Matty, and M. E. Smith, *Br. Med. J.*, **1,** 148 (1971).

39. M. B. Dahlke and E. Mertens-Roessler, *Blood*, **30,** 341 (1967).

40. C. D. Gerson, G. W. Hepner, N. Brown, N. Cohen, V. Herbert, and H. D. Janowitz, *Gastroenterology*, **63,** 246 (1972).

41. L. Elsborg, *Acta Haemat.*, **52,** 2 (1974).

42. D. Kelly, D. Weir, B. Reed, and J. Scott, *J. Clin. Invest.*, **64,** 1089 (1979).

43. C. L. Krumdieck, K. Fukushima, T. Fukushima, T. Shiota, and C. E. Butterworth, *Am. J. Clin. Nutr.*, **31,** 88 (1978).

44. M. Furlanut, P. Benetello, A. Avogaro, and R. Dainese, *Clin. Pharmacol. Ther.*, **24,** 294 (1978).

45. J. W. Norris and R. F. Pratt, *Drugs*, **8,** 366 (1974).

46. D. B. Smith and E. A. M. T. Obbens, in M. I. Botez and E. H. Reynolds, Eds., *Folic Acid in Neurology, Psychiatry, and Internal Medicine*, Raven, New York, 1979, pp. 267–283.

47. S. N. Wickramasinghe, *Clin. Lab. Haemat.*, **3,** 1 (1981).

48. R. Stebbins, J. Scott, and V. Herbert, *Semin. Hematol.*, **10**, 235 (1973).

49. D. W. Szeto, Y. Cheng, A. Rosowsky, C. Yu, E. J. Modest, J. R. Piper, R. D. Elliott, J. D. Rose and J. A. Montgomery, *Biochem. Pharmacol.*, **28**, 2633 (1979).

50. B. A. Kamen, P. A. Nylen, B. M. Camitta, and J. R. Bertino, *Brit. J. Haemat.*, **49**, 357 (1981).

51. N. L. Kobrinsky and N. K. C. Ramsay, *Ann. Intern. Med.*, **94**, 780 (1981).

52. J. Lindenbaum, N. Whitehead, and F. Reyner, *Am. J. Clin. Nutr.*, **28**, 346 (1975).

53. C. J. Paine, W. D. Grafton, V. L. Dickson, and E. R. Eichner, *Am. J. Clin. Nutr.*, **231**, 731 (1975).

54. R. J. West and J. K. Lloyd, *Gut*, **16**, 93 (1975).

55. G. H. Tomkin, D. R. Hadden, J. A. Weavers, and D. A. D. Montgomery, *Br. Med. J.*, **2**, 685 (1971).

56. G. H. Tomkin, *Br. Med. J.*, **3**, 673 (1973).

57. A. Coronato and G. B. J. Glass, *Proc. Soc. Exp. Biol. Med.*, **142**, 1341 (1973).

58. D. I. Webb, R. B. Chodos, C. Q. Mahar, and W. W. Faloon, *New Engl. J. Med.*, **279**, 845 (1968).

59. J. Lindenbaum and C. S. Lieber, *Nature*, **224**, 806 (1969).

60. E. D. Jacobson, R. B. Chodos, and W. W. Falcon, *Am. J. Med.*, **28**, 524 (1960).

61. O. Heinivara and I. P. Palva, *Acta Med. Scand.*, **177**, 337 (1965).

62. I. P. Palva, S. J. Salokannel, T. Timonen, and H. L. A. Palva, *Acta Med. Scand.*, **191**, 355 (1972).

63. C. H. Halsted and P. A. McIntyre, *Arch. Intern. Med.*, **130**, 935 (1972).

64. T. S. Callaghan, D. R. Hadden, and G. H. Tomkin, *Br. Med. J.*, **2**, 1214 (1980).

64a. V. Herbert and E. Jacob, *J. Am. Med. Assoc.*, **230**, 241 (1974).

65. H. L. Newmark, J. Scheiner, M. Marcus, and M. Prabhudesai, *Am. J. Clin. Nutr.*, **29**, 645 (1976).

66. V. Herbert, E. Jacob, K.-T. J. Wong, J. Scott, and R. D. Pfeffer, *Am. J. Clin. Nutr.*, **31**, 253 (1978).

67. S. Ekvall, I-W. Chen, and R. Bozian, *Am. J. Clin. Nutr.*, **34**, 1356 (1981).

68. J. J. Costanzi, B. K. Young, and R. Carmel, *Texas Rep. Biol. Med.*, 36, 69 (1978).

69. A. M. Shojania and B. Wylie, *Am. J. Obs. Gyn.*, 135, 129 (1979).

70. H. C. A. Lassen, E. Henriksen, F. Neukirch, and H. S. Kristensen, *Lancet*, **1**, 527 (1956).

71. H. C. A. Lassen and H. S. Kristensen, *Dan. Med. Bull.*, **6**, 252 (1959).

72. J. A. L. Amess, J. F. Burman, and D. L. Mollin, *Br. Med. J.*, **1**, 525 (1976).

73. J. A. L. Amess, J. F. Burman, G. M. Rees, D. G. Nancekievill, and D. L. Mollin, *Lancet*, **2**, 339 (1978).

74. R. B. Layzer, *Lancet*, **2**, 1227 (1978).

75. M. A. Nevins, *J. Am. Med. Assoc.*, **244**, 2264 (1980).

76. R. Deacon, M. Lumb, J. Perry, I. Chanarin, B. Minty, M. J. Halsy, and J. F. Nunn, *Lancet*, **2**, 1023 (1978).

77. H. Kondo, M. L. Osborne, J. F. Kolhouse, M. J. Binder, E. R. Podell, C. S. Utley, R. S. Abrams, and R. H. Allen, *J. Clin. Invest.*, **67**, 1270 (1981).

78. J. M. Scott and D. G. Weir, *Lancet*, **2**, 337 (1981).

79. J. M. Scott, J. H. Dinn, P. Wilson, and D. G. Weir, *Lancet*, **2**, 334 (1981).

6

Drugs in the Food Supply

SANFORD A. MILLER, Ph.D. and
JANE E. HARRIS, Ph.D.

Food and Drug Administration, Washington, D.C.

It is well accepted that the therapeutic or beneficial effects of drugs are often accompanied by undesirable, secondary effects. Specific side effects, which may be considered a nuisance by many of those taking the medication, may actually be life-threatening or produce irreversible damage (e.g., in teratogenesis) to a subpopulation whose medical status makes them uniquely sensitive to the drug. In view of these complicating factors, the physician, in effect, must perform a risk-benefit analysis for the patient before prescribing a particular drug to treat a medical condition. The physician is also expected to consider the medical status of the patient in advising him of what other medications are to be avoided, as well as to indicate the potential hazards associated with indulgence in such environmental toxins as alcohol and nicotine.

The use by the food industry of certain pharmacologically active substances as food additives has also been shown to have differential adverse effects on subpopulations, depending on the medical status inherent to that group. Although information about the potential side effects of food additives has been distributed to these subpopulations to some extent, control of exposure to a food additive is necessarily less than for a drug, in which a direct relationship between physician and patient exists. Of necessity, all of a population is potentially exposed to a food additive with little opportunity for selective restriction. As a result, the questions of whether substances pharmacologically active at or near use levels belong in the food supply as food additives, and to what extent the Food and Drug Administration should act to protect subpopulations demonstrating greater sensitivity to these products, are issues of increasing significance in today's world.

Although many known pharmacologically active substances are currently regulated as food additives, none is officially approved for its pharmacologic effects. Some are regulated for their flavoring properties (e.g., caffeine, methyl salicylate, quinine, ethanol) or for their intended physical effects, such as improvement of the solubility of component ingredients (e.g., diocyl sodium sulfosuccinate). Whereas at levels used for their flavoring properties or other intended effects few of these additives may produce biochemical or physiological effects, at least one—caffeine—may be added specifically for this purpose, although regulated on the basis of other functions. These effects may in general be considered desirable (such as the stimulant properties in the morning with caffeine) or, at other levels or under other conditions may be deleterious (such as the possible insomnia associated with caffeine exposure in the evening). Furthermore, increased sensitivity to the adverse effects of such pharmacologically active substances may exist in certain subpopulations. These subpopulations may include those of compromised medical status (e.g., debilitated elderly, hypertensive, and ulcerative patients, etc.), allergic individuals, as well as those of altered metabolic and physiologic states, such as the pregnant woman, the fetus, and the neonate. In this chapter we will limit the subpopulations under review to the fetus, neonate, and the young child in discussing and evaluating animal and epidemiologic studies that relate to the potential teratogenicity, reproductive toxicity, or behavioral effects associated with the food additives of one pharmacologically active substance—caffeine, in particular, and one other, methyl salicylate, as a comparison. The regulatory options currently available to the FDA for these substances and their legal limits will be addressed as will the problems inherent in providing safety to a minority of a population while assuring the rights of the majority.

Caffeine is a pharmacologically active substance that is a natural constitutent of the cola nut, coffee bean, and other materials. The current standard of identity for soda water characterizes "cola" and "pepper" type of soda as *requiring* caffeine and permits the addition of caffeine to any soda water at levels not to exceed 0.02% by weight in the finished drink. To an increasing extent, soda water beverages other than cola and pepper beverages contain caffeine as an optional ingredient in amounts equal to or greater than the amount of caffeine ordinarily present in the natural extract used in the flavoring of cola and pepper beverages. The addition of caffeine to soda water is permitted on the basis that caffeine was included in the 1959–1960 category of substances generally recognized as safe (GRAS), which was established by Congress when it enacted the Food Additives Amendment of 1958. The Flavor Extract Manufacturers' Association (FEMA) lists caffeine among the substances it considers to be GRAS for general use as a flavor, and it is on this basis that caffeine is currently being used on a limited basis as a flavoring agent in the nonbeverage food categories, including baked goods, frozen dairy desserts, gelatin puddings and fillings, and soft candy. Although used in other products, the predominant use of caffeine as an *added* ingredient is in soda water beverages, which accounts for the vast majority of the estimated two million pounds of caffeine added to food annually in the United States (this does not include the caffeine that occurs naturally in coffee, tea, cocoa, etc.).

The FDA's decision to place substances on the original GRAS lists of 1959-1960 was based on the data available at that time and on the state of knowledge in the field of toxicology. Since that time, new evidence has become available, patterns and levels of use have changed, and the state of the art in toxicology has advanced; all these factors have contributed to the Agency's decision to review and modify where appropriate these earlier determinations. To this end, the FDA initiated the GRAS review program in 1970. Under a contract, the Federation of American Societies for Experimental Biology (FASEB), acting through its Select Committee on GRAS Substances (SCOGS), compiled and evaluated the data and made recommendations to the Agency concerning the appropriate action to take on each substance. The 1978 FASEB report on caffeine recommended that caffeine in "cola-type beverages" should no longer be considered GRAS. FASEB placed primary emphasis on the behavioral effects of chronic exposure to caffeine in children during the period of brain growth and development. FASEB noted further that the estimated caffeine intake in children is near those levels that are known to cause central nervous system effects in adults. The FDA agrees with FASEB's concern about the addition to food of a pharmacologically active agent at levels that *may* produce behavioral effects, especially in young children. Furthermore, a recent teratology study performed at the FDA demonstrated teratogenic and fetotoxic effects of caffeine in rats at lower levels than have been previously reported. In view of these additional data, the potential behavioral, teratogenic, and reproductive effects of caffeine in humans were of sufficient concern to the FDA that additional studies have been proposed to resolve these questions. The effort to raise these issues and to assure performance of the necessary studies has led to a major political and legal debate and confrontation with the regulated industry. While these quasiscientific issues may be more exciting, this discussion of the scientific rationale behind FDA's concern about the food additive use of caffeine will be focused on the potential teratogenic, reproductive, and neurobehavioral effects of caffeine in the fetus, neonate, and young child.

The common sources of naturally occurring caffeine in foods such as coffee, tea, cocoa, and chocolate are listed in Table 1. It is interesting to

Table 1.   The Common Sources of Caffeine[a]

Product	Caffeine (mg)
Coffee	
Drip (5 oz)	146
Percolated (5 oz)	110
Instant, regular (5 oz)	53
Decaffeinated (5 oz)	2
Tea	
One-minute brew (5 oz)	9 to 33
Three-minute brew (5 oz)	20 to 46
Five-minute brew (5 oz)	20 to 50
Canned ice tea (12 oz)	22 to 36
Cocoa and chocolate	
Cocoa beverage (water mix, 6 oz)	10
Milk chocolate (1 oz)	6
Baking chocolate (1 oz)	35

[a] From *Consumer Reports*.

note that varying the method of preparing coffee, i.e., drip vs. perco-
lated vs. instant, leads to decreased levels of caffeine from 150 to 110 to
50 mg/cup. Similarly, increasing the brewing time of tea from one mi-
nute to five minutes elevates the caffeine concentration from 9 to 50 mg.
Another significant source of naturally occurring caffeine is the cola nut,
which is employed in the manufacture of cola and pepper soda waters.
Approximately 35 to 45 mg of caffeine are present in most colas and
peppers. Perhaps more important, caffeine is added to products where
it is not traditionally found. Many of the newer soft drinks, mostly citrus
based, contained increasingly higher levels of caffeine—up to 52 mg/12
oz. As a result soft drinks have become a major source of caffeine for
children of all ages. Estimates of caffeine consumption from coffee, tea,
or soda waters at all age levels for high-intake populations are presented
in Table 2. An adult consuming six cups of regular coffee a day would
have a daily intake of about 15 mg/kg body weight, or 30 mg/kg at 12
cups/day. An adult noncoffee drinker who consumes six cans of soda
water would have a daily intake of 4 mg/kg body weight. A child weigh-
ing 30 kg (seven to ten years old) may consume as much as a glass of iced
tea and two cans of soda water with an estimated total intake of 4 mg/kg/
day. A 15 kg child (three year old), ingesting one-half this amount of
beverage, on a body weight basis would consume a similar level, i.e., 4

Table 2.   Caffeine Consumption

Age	Coffee (C) or Tea (T), 150 mg/cup (C) or 30 mg/cup (T)		Soda Water 40 mg/12 oz can		Total mg/kg/day
Adult (60 kg)	6 (C) cups	15 mg/kg/day	6 cans	4 mg/kg/day	4-15
Child (30 kg)	1 (T) cup	1 mg/kg/day	2 cans	3 mg/kg/day	4
Young child (15 kg)	1/1 (T) cup	1 mg/kg/day	1 can	3 mg/kg/day	4
Neonate (3 kg)	Lactation (level in milk up to 7 mg/l)		150 ml milk/kg		1

mg/kg/day. Finally, studies have shown concentrations of caffeine in the milk of the lactating mother to be twice the maternal plasma concentrations. Assays of maternal milk for caffeine have demonstrated levels up to 7 mg/liter and assuming consumption by the neonate of 150 ml of milk/kg body weight, the total intake of caffeine for the neonate may be as much as 1 mg/kg/day.

To predict the pharmacological effects of caffeine, knowledge of the consumption level or dose is important as are the pharmacokinetic parameters, specifically the rates of metabolism and excretion. The influence of age or physiological condition on the plasma half-life of caffeine is shown in Table 3. Recent studies suggest that the six- to ten-year-old child actually eliminates caffeine at twice the rate of adults. The premature infant and neonate, however, have not developed the enzymatic ca-

Table 3.   Elimination of Caffeine

Condition or Age	Half-Life (Plasma) $t_{1/2}$ (hr)
Adult	5–6
Child (6–10 yrs)	2–3
Premature and newborn infants	98
7–9 mo infant	4
Pregnancy	
1–3 mo (1st trimester)	6
4–9 mo (2nd to 3rd trimesters)	10–18
1 wk postpartum	6
Oral contraceptive use	12
Smokers	3.5

pacity necessary for metabolizing caffeine; this, in addition to the neonate's compromised ability for excreting compounds, results in a half-life of four days in the neonate, a value 16 times longer than in the adult. By seven to nine months, this capacity to metabolize and excrete caffeine reaches the adult level. The endocrine changes associated with pregnancy appear to slow the metabolism of caffeine, in addition to many other drugs. An increase in the plasma half-life from six to ten hours is first observed in the second trimester at four months, and by the third trimester increases to 18 hours, which is three times longer than nonpregnant rates. The capacity to metabolize caffeine returns to normal by the first week postpartum. A similar influence of the endocrine system on the P-450 mixed-function oxidase system involved in caffeine metabolism is shown by the prolonged half-life associated with the use of oral contraceptives. In contrast, smoking appears to induce the cytochrome P-450 system and increase the rate of caffeine metabolism. These differences in ability to metabolize and excrete caffeine are important in assessing the potential developmental toxicity of caffeine in the fetus, neonate, and young child.

The results of a recent teratology study performed by Dr. T. X. Collins and his associates at the FDA in which rats were orally intubated with caffeine at doses from 6 to 125 mg/kg body weight/day are presented in Table 4. The lowest dose producing statistically significant increases in malformations and fetal death was at 80 mg/kg body weight/day. These teratogenic effects included ectrodactyly (missing digits) and resorptions. It should be noted that at the 80 mg/kg/day dose, significant maternal toxicity was evident (as observed by decreased food consumption and weight gain). On the other hand, ectrodactyly has not been reported previously in pregnant animals in which decreased food intake and weight gain were induced by other means. Retarded growth (an increase

Table 4.   Developmental Toxicity of Caffeine

Effect	Lowest Effect Dose (LED) mg/kg/day/Rat	LED mg/kg/day Human
Teratogenic		
Ectrodactyly	80	?
Resorptions	80	
Retarded growth	40	
Delay in skeletal ossification		
of sternebrae	40	?

in runts and decrease in fetal weights), as well as delays in skeletal ossification of the sternebrae were observed in the 40 mg/kg/day dose group; the delay in skeletal ossification is difficult to interpret since it is often found to be transient.

Teratogenic effects and developmental toxicity have not been definitively associated with caffeine consumption in humans in the available epidemiology studies, all of which, unfortunately, have methodological problems resulting from inadequate control for such confounding variables as smoking, age of mother, alcohol, genetic predisposition, or other drug use. Unfavorable outcomes of pregnancy that might be related to insults to fetal development may include spontaneous abortion, congenital malformation, stillbirth and infant mortality, low birth weight (prematurity or in utero growth restriction), and retarded infant development, which may be physiological or behavioral in nature. In the absence of adequate direct epidemiologic investigations on caffeine with respect to its potential for producing congenital defects and other unfavorable pregnancy outcomes, caffeine doses associated with developmental toxicity in the rat can be related to that of human consumption and plasma half-lives (Table 5). Malformations or congenital defects, as well as spontaneous abortions, generally occur in the human during the first trimester of pregnancy when the capacity to metabolize caffeine is still normal. On the other hand, alterations in the size and weight of the fetus are more readily influenced by in utero conditions of the third trimester. In consideration of fetal growth, the plasma half-life of caffeine is prolonged to 18 hours in the third trimester, thereby subjecting the fetus to higher levels of caffeine in utero. This elevated exposure of the fetus to caffeine would increase the likelihood of potential growth-retarding ef-

Table 5. Developmental Toxicity of Caffeine

Effect	LED mg/kd/day (Rat)	Human Consumption mg/kg/day	Human Plasma $t_{1/2}$ (hr)
Malformations	80	4–15	6 (1st trimester)
Resorptions	80	4–15	6 (1st trimester)
Reduced fetal size and weights	40	4–15	18 (3rd trimester)
Delay in skeletal ossification	40	4–15	18 (3rd trimester)
Retarded infant develoment	?	1 (nursing neonate)	98 1–3 mo postpartum)

fects of caffeine, which are observed in the rat at a bolus dose of 40 mg/kg. A delay in skeletal ossification, which was also observed at the dose of 40 mg/kg in the rat, is difficut to extrapolate to the human because much variability has been observed at birth in the degree of ossification. We do not yet know the long-term sequelae on bone development of such delays in development. Finally, the nursing neonate, who may be exposed on a daily basis to as much as 1 mg/kg/day, demonstrates a compromised capacity to metabolize and excrete caffeine (about 1/16 that of an older infant) and, as a result, would be subjected over a prolonged period to significantly elevated plasma levels of caffeine. However, by nine months of age, the infant has developed the enzymatic activity observed in the adult for metabolizing caffeine. This exposure of the nursing neonate to high plasma levels of caffeine could possibly contribute in part to disturbances in the sleep patterns of the neonate and consequently in those of the parents as well!

The long-term neurobehavioral effects resulting from the exposure of the developing nervous system to high levels of caffeine are difficult to predict. Nevertheless, it is possible to enumerate both positive and negative consequences of acute or chronic consumption of caffeine in children and adults. Positive effects include improved motor performance, decreased fatigue, enhanced sensory activity, and increased alertness. These positive effects may partly explain the predilection, bordering on compulsion, for a majority of adults to consume coffee, tea, or soft drinks in the morning ritual of awakening. In contrast, negative responses have also been reported with caffeine at levels that vary in accordance with the sensitivity of the individual and the degree of tolerance which develops during chronic exposure. These responses include irritability, nervousness or anxiety, tremor, jitteriness and jumpiness in children, headache, insomnia, and withdrawal headaches. These responses have been reported (Table 6) to occur at doses as low as 2 to 4 mg/kg in the adult and 10 mg/kg in ten-year-old children, with unknown but presumably lower effective dose levels in the neonate. Studies in mice show increases in motor activity and changes in discriminatory be-

Table 6. Neurobehavioral Effects of Caffeine

Effect	LED mg/kg/day Mouse	LED mg/kg/day Human
Motor activity	1–2	2–3 (Adult)
Discrimination		10 (10-yr-old child)
		? (Neonate)

Table 7. Neurobehavioral Effects of Caffeine in Humans

Condition or Age	LED mg/kg/day	Consumption mg/kg/day	Plasma $t_{1/2}$ (hr)
Adult	2–4	4–15	5–6
Child (10 yrs)	10	4	2–3
Neonate (nursing)	?	1	98
Fetus (2nd or 3rd trimester)	?	4–15	10–18

havior at acute doses as low as 1 to 2 mg/kg. The relationship in humans of the lowest stimulatory doses to the high consumption levels and plasma half-lives for caffeine is shown in Table 7. One might note that in comparison with the adult, the higher effect level for the two-year-old child may be related to the shorter plasma half-life of caffeine. In contrast, the half-life of caffeine, which is 16 times longer in the neonate than in the adult, may make the newborn particularly sensitive to even low levels of caffeine consumed in the mother's milk. Finally, the fetus, which relies on the maternal capacity to metabolize caffeine, would be exposed to two to three times higher levels of caffeine in the second and third trimester than in the first trimester, based on the slower rate of metabolizing caffeine late in pregnancy. Thus, the exposure to high levels of caffeine through the maternal circulation and lactation may present an increased risk situation to the fetus and neonate, especially in view of the continuing formation of synaptic dendritic proliferation and axonal extention in the developing central nervous system in utero and in postnatal life.

Another very old flavoring agent used in foods is methyl salicylate, or oil of wintergreen. Concern about the food additive use of methyl salicylate arose in 1959 and the early 1960s when reports showed that the administration of high doses of methyl salicylate in test animals resulted in an increased incidence of cardiovascular and skeletal malformations. These teratogenic doses are at least a 100 times greater than the levels associated with the food additive use of salicylates. Thus, it appears that the weak teratogenic potential of salicylates in test animals indicates a low risk for the human consuming methyl salicylate as a flavoring agent.

The FDA has taken responsibility to see that questions raised about the potential neurobehavioral effects and developmental toxicity of caffeine be investigated to protect the rights of the majority to a safe food supply. During this investigatory period, the FDA has proposed that the uses of caffeine be restricted to current uses and levels and that the presence of caffeine as an added ingredient be reflected on the label to in-form pregnant women and mothers of young children who want to curb or avoid caffeine-containing foods that the product contains caffeine. In addition, the Commissioner has initiated a program to provide the public with information concerning the possible adverse effects of caffeine, especially in pregnancy. The FDA has also questioned the *purpose* of adding caffeine to foods, especially soft drinks, at levels demonstrated to have stimulatory effects on the central nervous system. Although it is unclear whether the FDA has authority under the law to prohibit the use of a food ingredient solely because the ingredient is a stimulant, the indiscriminate use of any pharmacologically active substance as a food ingredient at levels approximating the pharmacologic effect raises serious public health questions, especially where, as in the case of caffeine, the foods involved are consumed widely by children.

Several important points can be derived from the preceding discussion. First, although there is no question that caffeine is an animal teratogen, it must be noted that there is no evidence thus far that the consumption of caffeine by humans has, in general, produced any deleterious effect. As indicated earlier, a comprehensive review of all the available epidemiological data by an interagency committee of epidemiologists concluded that there were no studies of sufficient power or sufficiently unflawed that could be used to determine the potential for human harm of caffeine. Thus the question remains open, and indeed, several other major issues need to be resolved before the question of caffeine's role in the etiology of human birth defects, among other possible deleterious effects, can be determined. We do not know, for example, whether the models used for experimental teratogenesis can be translated to human experience; i.e., we do not understand the process of experimental teratogenesis sufficiently to enable us to make reasonable assumptions on potential human harm from the process. Second, we are unable to translate the fact of caffeine's central nervous system effects to the problem of possible human harm, particularly in reference to the effect of caffeine on the developing nervous system. In this case, our models are so crude and insensitive that we are not certain if these models are measuring important behavioral and central nervous system effects. For example, very recent and very preliminary unpublished data suggest that caffeine may act as a type of "chemical conditioner or primer" for audiogenic responses in mice. In experiments in which normal mice, not having a genetic or audiogenic lesion, were exposed to caffeine early in the postnatal period and then at some later time exposed to audiogenic stimuli, caffeine was shown to increase significantly the audiogenic response of these animals. The meaning of this finding and its mechanism are as yet unknown. However, the data suggest that there may be effects of substances such as caffeine that are only inferred and have not yet been specifically determined. Further, the meaning of this finding in terms of public health and more specifically the regulatory action that might be taken by agencies such as FDA are largely unknown. Third, irrespective of the findings of potential harm from the use of substances such as caffeine, we are still faced with the ethical question of whether it is appropriate to add to foods substances having known pharmacological effects specifically for those effects. Food occupies a particularly sensitive place in our culture. To add known pharmacological agents to the food supply without the specific, conscious decision of the consumer can be an ethical problem. Finally, there still remains the question of what regulatory strategies can be used for substances such as caffeine that affect only segments of the population. Traditionally, national regulatory strategies are based on the assumption that the potential harm is spread more or less evenly across the entire population. Thus the question of risk becomes a statistical problem that can theoretically be deduced from a variety of data. On the other hand, there are no simple regulatory strategies when only a segment of the population is affected because of age, physiologic state, or genetic susceptibility. Until now, the only tools available to regulatory agencies to deal with these problems were labeling or public information. The use of the label is limited by its small size and by the fact that a continual series of warnings on the label reduces their impact. Similarly, public education programs suffer from overuse. It seems clear that more thought must be given to the development of new regulatory theories that consider this question of protecting the rights of the majority, while at the same time considering the needs of the minority. In the end, however, the lack of a good scientific base to allow isolation of the issues of ethics and law from those of science is perhaps the greatest weakness in the solution of the problem. Unfortunately, the development of new research strategies in response to these scientific questions is occurring at a time when national fiscal policy has made the funding of this research more difficult. It is hoped that in the planning for and in the establishment of national research priorities, these issues are recognized as being among the most important for our society today. Without the necessary scientific base for discussion, no rational national policy for their resolution can be developed.

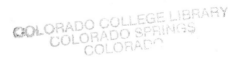

7

Lipid-Lowering Drugs and Low-Fat Diets

ROBERT H. PALMER, M.D.

Columbia University College of Physicians and Surgeons, New York, New York

There is considerable interest in the role of cholesterol and other lipids in the pathogenesis of arteriosclerosis, and there is considerable controversy over the use of low-fat diets and lipid-lowering drugs for the prevention of arteriosclerosis. Why should this be, and what are we to conclude about the proper role of these therapies?

ROLE OF LIPIDS IN ARTERIOSCLEROSIS

There are six major risk factors for coronary artery disease (CAD). The first might be termed dyslipidemia, or dyslipoproteinemia. The initial association was made with elevated serum cholesterol levels, but it is now clear that a variety of lipid disturbances predispose to CAD. Hypercholesterolemia, the major form of dyslipidemia, is one of the three main remediable risk factors, the other two being hypertension and cigarette smoking. The next three risk factors, diabetes, a type-A personality, and a strong family history of CAD, are increasingly *less* amenable to intervention.

In addition to the major risk factors, a number of others have been shown to be of importance in either clinical or animal studies: obesity; sedentary life style; a diet low in alcohol, fiber, or minerals or high in sucrose or animal protein; disorders of cysteine metabolism; estrogen administration; vasectomy; and many others. Because many of these

Supported in part by grant # HL 21006, Specialized Center of Research (SCOR) in Arteriosclerosis, National Heart, Lung and Blood Institute.

have a number of physiological consequences, it is not clear whether they are independent risk factors or whether they influence risk through effects on other primary factors.

Serum lipids and lipoproteins act to promote atherogenesis in several ways. The association of total serum cholesterol with CAD has been shown to be due largely to the low density lipoprotein (LDL) cholesterol. The major steps in that process have now been worked out using the genetic disorder of familial hypercholesterolemia. LDL cholesterol elevations from other causes are also atherogenic, and there is some evidence that elevated levels of apoprotein B may predispose to atherosclerosis even in the presence of relatively normal LDL cholesterol.

A relation between elevated triglycerides and arteriosclerosis, first demonstrated in epidemiological studies, has not been found in some studies in which the covariance of triglycerides with HDL cholesterol has been considered. Nevertheless there are some who feel that elevated triglycerides still constitute a risk factor for some patients—particularly those with problems in remnant clearance.

Recently much attention has been given to HDL cholesterol, and it is clear that a low level of HDL cholesterol, particularly the HDL_2 subclass, is a powerful predictor of increased risk even in the absence of elevated triglycerides.

Finally, an unusual but easily treatable lipid disorder is the "Type III" remnant disease, characterized by the accumulation of cholesterol-rich very low density lipoproteins (VLDL) and due to the absence of a specific isoform of the E apoprotein that apparently facilitates hepatic removal of these particles. Thus there is a whole family of disturbances of lipoprotein metabolism that is associated with increased risk of CAD.

The rationale for treating elevated lipids is based on the lipid hypothesis. This hypothesis was based on data such as that from the Framingham study, which showed that the risk of CAD increases with increasing cholesterol level, and that this holds true for all levels of cholesterol—though the relation is stronger at higher levels and in the presence of other risk factors. The hypothesis is that if the cholesterol level is reduced, the risk will also be reduced. For HDL cholesterol, of course, the shape of the curve would be reversed, but the same rationale would apply. Of course, this is obviously a hypothesis because other factors could conceivably alter both risk and serum cholesterol independently without implying causality.

It has proved extremely difficult to test the lipid hypothesis adequately for a variety of reasons. The most important is that it has been difficult to make major changes in serum lipid levels in humans. Some of the better studies of dietary intervention have achieved reductions of

15%, but most drug studies have achieved reductions of under 10%. In fact, we can be sure that an adequate dietary study will never be done because a special commission, a few years ago, reviewed the question in detail and concluded that an adequate trial would not be feasible. Drug studies can be run more effectively, and, though they are difficult and cumbersome, several are in progress or have been completed recently. In particular, the recent WHO study of clofibrate has provided some of the first compelling evidence that lowering cholesterol can prevent heart attacks. In that study, the heart attack rates in a high-cholesterol control group, a high-cholesterol group treated with clofibrate, and a low-cholesterol control group were related to the serum cholesterol levels during the trial in a manner very reminiscent of the Framingham data. In another type of study, a group of patients with documented femoral arteriosclerosis was treated intensively with diet, hypolipidemic drugs, and antihypertensive medications. There was a clear difference in serum lipid changes between the group in whom the disease progressed and the group in whom it regressed. When clinical data of this type are combined with data from animal studies, it seems highly probable that decreasing serum lipids can mitigate the progression of arteriosclerosis. We can be relatively confident about recommending reduction of LDL cholesterol for the prevention of CAD. It should be noted, however, that there have been *no* intervention trials aimed at elevating HDL levels, and so the value of intervening to raise HDL levels remains hypothetical at this time. Before concluding that interventions that raise or lower HDL levels have an effect on CAD, we need to know more about the *mechanism* by which HDL appears to protect, and whether the effect is restricted to certain species of HDL that may move in different directions during different interventions. We have learned from the LDL/HDL story that superficial conclusions based on total levels may prove to be erroneous when subgroups are considered.

EVALUATING THE NEED FOR TREATMENT

If we conclude that elevated LDL cholesterol is a risk factor and that lowering LDL cholesterol will reduce risk, who should be treated? To answer that question we have to consider first what is a normal and what is an abnormal cholesterol value.

The first problem is that we start by relating total (and LDL) cholesterol levels to those of the general population. By tradition we say that values above the 95th percentile are abnormal. But cholesterol levels increase with age, so that we have to construct separate tables for different age groups. Then women have lower cholesterol values prior to menopause and higher values after, so that additional tables are needed. Women taking contraceptives require still another table, and if other factors affecting cholesterol levels were taken into consideration a whole series of tables would be necessary to cover a myriad of subgroups. As it is, the 95th percentile varies from about 216 to over 300 mg/dl.

A more important problem with percentiles is that they do not have any specific biological relevance. Epidemiological studies show that there is no abrupt change in risk at the 95th percentile, but there is a smooth, progressive increase in risk with increasing cholesterol. Thus, a person at the 50th percentile in the country might be at greater risk than one at the 90th percentile in a low-risk population. So it is probably an oversimplification to speak of normal and abnormal levels when we should be looking at a given level as reflecting *relative* risk. The *absolute* risk can not be predicted for a given level as it is influenced first by other risk factors and second (which may be a variation on the same theme) by the particular ability of the individual to tolerate elevated cholesterol levels.

The same logic holds for HDL levels. They do not vary with age, but in addition to being different in men and women, they are influenced by a variety of factors including activity, smoking, alcohol, and various drugs. Whether variations related to these parameters are associated with changes in risk remains to be seen.

Parenthetically, the mechanism by which HDL levels appear to protect against CAD is unknown. It has been thought that HDL might act to remove cholesterol from tissues, but recent studies in our laboratory have failed to demonstrate a relation between total body cholesterol and HDL levels. Perhaps the effect of HDL will have more to do with prostaglandin metabolism and vessel wall function.

Based on these considerations, a scheme for the evaluation and treatment of hyperlipidemia can be developed. First, the patient's total risk status should be evaluated. The evaluation should include determinations of the type and severity of dyslipidemia (elevation of LDL, reductions in HDL). Second, causes of secondary hyperlipidemia, if any, should be sought and corrected. Third, a feasible nutritional program should be instituted and the results evaluated. Finally, depending on the results of dietary interventions, drug therapy should be considered. If it is instituted, it should be monitored and evaluated. At each stage, the benefits and disadvantages have to be considered as they pertain to the individual patient.

DIETARY TREATMENT OF HYPERLIPIDEMIA

The objectives in dietary treatment of hyperlipidemia are to decrease body weight, because of the many ways that obesity adversely effects lipid metabolism, to decrease serum cholesterol and thereby LDL levels, and to decrease serum triglycerides. The last is more because elevated triglyceride levels are indicative of disturbances in lipid metabolism than because of any innate atherogenicity. For example, decreasing serum triglycerides may result in a rise in serum HDL levels.

The means whereby these objectives are accomplished include restrictions of calories, saturated fat, cholesterol, and refined carbohydrate, and more liberal use of polyunsaturated fat and complex carbohydrates. Of these, the primary emphasis should be on restriction of saturated fat (which is the source of a large portion of the calories and cholesterol in the diet) with replacement by complex carbohydrates and less-saturated fat as necessary. There is a growing consensus behind the guidelines recommended by the American Heart Association as the initial approach to the treatment of most forms of hyperlipidemia. These restrict saturated fat to less than 10% of total calories and permit 10% of calories from monounsaturates and 10% from polyunsaturates.

Restriction of cholesterol to less than 300 mg/day is recommended. Aside from eggs, liver, and obvious fat in beef, cream, and dairy products, there is not as much variation in cholesterol content of foods as some people imagine. Nevertheless, to maintain an intake of under 300 mg/day requires attention to these differences. For severe forms of hyperlipidemia, more severe restriction of cholesterol intake or other modifications may be recommended.

What can be expected from dietary manipulation? The results depend on both sociological and biological factors. Under metabolic ward conditions, reductions of 30% in cholesterol are perfectly feasible. In clinical trials, using regular food, a 15% reduction is a reasonable target. In community studies, without the intense effort in compliance, 7% may be a more realistic estimate—depending on the motivation of the individuals or groups involved.

In addition to problems of compliance, there are biological differences in the way individuals adapt to changes in cholesterol intake. Some patients respond to increased intake by decreasing their own synthesis in a compensatory fashion, while others accumulate cholesterol. Of these some increase their plasma levels while others do not—and sequester cholesterol in various tissues.

The implication of all this is that some people are likely to benefit from reducing their cholesterol intake whereas others are not. Unfortunately, we have no way of predicting who will respond, so we must rely on individual clinical trials, monitoring the response of each patient. Even this will not allow us to determine what is going on in tissues; some patients accumulate cholesterol with no increase in plasma cholesterol whereas others do not accumulate cholesterol despite increases in plasma cholesterol. So recommendations concerning dietary intervention rest on reasoning and a certain amount of direct and circumstantial evidence. Of course, they may be modified by a variety of factors—including personal value judgments.

In attempting to evaluate the costs and benefits of dietary intervention it is important to remember that these are all conditional. The benefits to be expected depend first on the risk status of the individual, including lipid factors such as LDL level and HDL level, as well as other risk factors. Second, they depend on the extent of reduction that can be achieved, which depends in turn on what the person's habitual diet is, how much a change he or she is willing to make, and whether he or she is biologically responsive. Similarly, the costs, in terms of effort and possible changes in quality of life, depend on how great a restriction is being contemplated, on what individual, family, and societal pressures exist to interfere with compliance, and on whether dietary modifications may turn out to have unanticipated effects.

We are left, then, with some major questions about the dietary treatment of hyperlipidemia. The scientific question of whether it will reduce mortality and morbidity probably never will be answered conclusively, but the bulk of evidence suggests that it will—at least for some groups of people. There is a more difficult philosophical question; for whom should dietary intervention be recommended? Some people stand to benefit more than others, but I submit that most people stand to benefit to a greater or lesser extent. If so, who should make such a recommendation? Ideally, each person should have his risk status assessed and receive an appropriate recommendation. Practically, it makes sense for organizations such as the American Heart Association to make recommendations (in a country such as ours with high cholesterol levels and high rates of CAD) to the country as a whole, recognizing that unncessary changes may be made by a few as part of a movement to provide a climate in which changes can and will be made by the majority who really do stand to benefit. This raises the final political question of the role of government. Can the government be effective in changing the eating patterns of the country, and if so, should it engage in such an activity? The answers to these questions are difficult and important. Failure to deal with them directly has led to controversial recommendations, charges, and countercharges.

DRUG TREATMENT OF HYPERLIPIDEMIA

Leaving dietary treatment, which should be the first step in any treatment program, let us turn briefly to the question of drug treatment. Everything that has been said about the individual's risk status on the one hand and the risks and benefits of treatment on the other, applies equally to drug treatment—except that the risks and disadvantages of drugs tend to be greater.

The mainstay of treatment for hypercholesterolemia is the resins, colestipol and cholestyramine. They act to enhance hepatic uptake of LDL, as a result of their interruption of the enterohepatic circulation of bile acids. Side effects, though occasionally bothersome, are not serious and consist mainly of constipation and miscellaneous gastrointestinal symptoms. The resins may bind certain drugs, with obvious consequences, and marked elevation of serum triglycerides occasionally occurs in patients with hypertriglyceridemia.

Clofibrate is one of the most extensively studied drugs in the world, and the only one so far conclusively shown to decrease the rate of myocardial infarctions. The mechanism of action is controversial but may include decreased VLDL production as well as increased VLDL catabolism and enhanced cholesterol secretion in bile. It is excreted by the kidneys, so the dose must be reduced in renal failure.

The major adverse effect of clofibrate is an eightfold increase in the incidence of cholelithiasis. For reasons that are probably not related to the drug, mortality in the treated group was increased in the WHO study; however the possibility that the diffuse increase in mortality *may* have been related to the drug has caused the FDA to impose restrictions on its distribution. It is, unfortunately, unlikely that this will be clarified further. There are a number of other side effects to this drug, but it should be noted that its use in patients with hypertriglyceridemia may result in elevations in LDL by enhancing the catabolism of VLDL.

Probucol is a drug that lowers LDL but not VLDL levels. However, it also lowers HDL levels, and this has raised concern over whether the total effect is beneficial or not. We have discussed the problem of interpreting changes in HDL earlier, but regardless of this effect on HDL, the drug has been shown to be effective in reducing xanthomata and there have been some impressive regression studies in animal models. Probucol is quite well tolerated and is convenient to take.

Nicotinic acid (*not* nicotinamide) is currently being used extensively. It is a potent drug, when used in 4–6 g amounts, with a number of advantages and disadvantages. It is particularly effective in lowering LDL cholesterol when used in conjunction with high doses of the resins, and decreases over 50% can be seen in the usually intractable heterozygous familial hypercholesterolemia. It is also the only medication, other than clofibrate, to lower serum triglycerides, and it is one of the very few that clearly raise HDL cholesterol. On the other hand, the doses must be increased gradually to prevent hepatotoxicity. Flushing, which can be quite intense, is frequently a problem, though it can be minimized by taking one aspirin tablet 1/2 hour before the dose. It should be taken after meals to decrease gastric irritation. Its effect on blood glucose and uric acid may pose problems for patients with diabetes or gout.

Finally, there are several ancillary agents that may be useful. β-sitosterol, given as 30 ml of plant sterols before meals and at bedtime, reduces cholesterol absorption and produces modest cholesterol lowering. Its main side effect, a mild laxative one, makes it convenient to use with the resins. It is moderately expensive.

Neomycin is cheap and well tolerated. It is mainly not absorbed and creates insoluble complexes with bile salts as well as altering the bacterial flora of the large bowel. Very rarely, particularly in renal disease, the small amounts that may be absorbed can accumulate and cause serious renal or 8th nerve damage.

D-thyroxine is also cheap and easy to take. Its main side effect is a thyroxine-like dose-dependent hypermetabolism, so that in secondary clinical trials its use has been associated with increased mortality due to arrhythmias (in the context of a diseased myocardium). Some feel that it is a very useful drug in young people when one can be confident there is not pre-existing coronary disease.

Finally, para-aminosalicylic acid apparently is effective in lowering LDL and VLDL, but earlier preparations were associated with frequent gastrointestinal side effects. A newer formulation, PAS-C, is said to be better tolerated, but there is little clinical information about it and it is not widely used.

In summary, disorders of lipid metabolism are one of several major risk factors for coronary artery disease. Hypercholesterolemia together with smoking and hypertension constitute the major factors amenable to risk factor intervention. The physician is faced with a patient population in which the risk for CAD varies over a wide range. The physician also has available a good series of interventions, from modest dietary restriction alone to severe restriction plus multiple drugs. Each of these interventions entails risks and benefits that must be weighed against the risk of the disease. In that process the patient and physician must weigh facts and prejudices, as well as philosophical and practical considerations.

8

Effect of Diet and Sulfonylurea Drugs on Insulin Resistance and Insulin-Receptor Function

F. XAVIER PI-SUNYER, M.D.

Columbia University College of Physicians and Surgeons New York, New York

Any discussion of dietary or drug effects on diabetes mellitus and insulin action today must include a review of insulin receptors and their function. Insulin is secreted from the beta cell of the pancreas and courses as a free peptide in the blood stream until it attaches to cells. The now classic studies of Roth and his colleagues (1) have shown that the first step in the action of insulin on the cell is the binding of the hormone to a specific receptor on the outer plasma membrane. The combining of the hormone with the receptor then initiates a series of steps on the membrane and/or the cell interior which lead to a variety of postreceptor events, among them: (1) stimulation of membrane transport of sugars, amino acids, ions such as potassium, and nucleotide precursors, (2) activation and inhibition of both membrane-bound and soluble enzymes, (3) stimulation of protein synthesis, (4) inhibition of protein degradation, (5) stimulation of messenger DNA and RNA synthesis, and (6) alteration of cell morphology.

The nature of the postreceptor events (that is, steps beyond the initial binding between hormone and receptor) that generate these multifaceted responses in target cells are not known, although important information on the biochemistry of the process is being elucidated. It is now evident, however, that the number of surface insulin receptors on a cell is a major factor in the responsiveness of the given cell to insulin

The author is particularly indebted to the authors of Refs. 1 and 8 for use of their information in the preparation of this manuscript.

(1,2). In certain disease states, a decreased number of insulin receptors leads to insulin insensitivity. Generally, where high levels of insulin prevail in the blood, low levels of insulin receptors are present. This self-regulation of the membrane insulin receptor, so that high insulin levels cause a lowering of insulin-receptor number, has been called down-regulation, and it has been demonstrated both in vivo (3) and in vitro on cells in culture (4).

Changes in numbers of receptors and in insulin binding have been described after certain dietary programs and after treatment with certain sulfonylurea antidiabetic drugs. It is the purpose of this chapter to review the changes in insulin receptors and postreceptor function occurring in cells of diabetic and obese subjects who have been treated with diet or with oral antidiabetic sulfonylurea drugs.

OBESITY AND INSULIN RESISTANCE

Since many non-insulin-dependent (Type 2) diabetic subjects are obese, the influence of obesity on insulin resistance and insulin-receptor and postreceptor function will be discussed first. Obesity has long been known to induce an insulin-resistant state in man (5–7). Recent investigation has attributed part of this resistance to changes in insulin-receptor number and/or receptor affinity for insulin and part of it to postreceptor defects.

Insulin resistance can be caused by decreased insulin sensitivity or decreased insulin responsiveness. Decreased insulin sensitivity is defined as a decrease in the proportion of the total hormonal response that occurs at any given submaximal concentration of insulin (8). That is, with decreased sensitivity, the concentration of insulin required to produce a given submaximal response to insulin by the cell will be greater. While the dose-response curve will shift towards the right, so that higher concentrations of hormone will be required to produce a given effect, high enough concentration of insulin will produce the same maximal response (9).

Decreased insulin responsiveness is an impairment in the maximal effect of insulin on the particular insulin action under study (8). If a maximal response is not produced, decreased insulin responsiveness occurs. Since only about 10% of insulin receptors have to be occupied to produce a maximum biological effect (10), if enough receptors are occupied and the maximal effect is not attained, a step distal to the insulin receptor must be defective. Even if receptor number is decreased, with a high enough insulin concentration the critical number of receptors should be filled to allow a maximal response, and defective responsiveness then implies a postreceptor defect (8).

The insulin target cells most often used for studies of insulin binding have been adipocytes, monocytes, or hepatocytes because these are the more easily obtained and prepared cells from animals or human volunteers. More recently, erythrocytes have also been used and results have been similar to those obtained with more traditional insulin target cells. Although adipocytes and hepatocytes clearly are target cells for insulin, the role of insulin in monocytes and erythrocytes has been less clear, though insulin does affect two specific immune functions of murine monocyte-like cells (11,12). It now seems clear that cells from obese men (13–16) and obese animals (3,17–20) have a decreased number of insulin receptors.

The insulin resistance of obesity has been extensively studied in animal models of obesity. Both the ob/ob and the db/db mouse show a resistance that is characterized by a decreased number of insulin receptors (17,19,21,22). These mice are hyperinsulinemic, hyperglycemic, and insulin resistant. Although it is likely that the sequence of events leads from hyperphagia to hyperglycemia, to hyperinsulinemia, to decreased insulin receptors, it is possible that the initial lesion is decreased insulin receptors and that the hyperinsulinemia and hyperglycemia follow (1).

Although Soll et al. (19) proposed a decrease in the number of receptor sites as a generalized mechanism for cellular insulin resistance, this has not been borne out by later investigation. In fact, it has become clear that the tissues of obese animal models show intracellular postreceptor defects in glucose metabolism which account for the major part of insulin resistance (20,23–27).

Because it is difficult to extrapolate from animal in vitro tissue studies and/or in vivo studies to the human insulin-resistant obese state, investigations have been extended to man. The overall in vivo dose-response curve of normal and obese subjects was studied by measuring glucose disposal at a number of steady-state plasma concentrations of insulin and showed a shift to the right in the response curve (16), suggesting that decreased insulin receptors contributed to the insulin-resistant state. But the degree of insulin resistance was much greater than could be predicted from the magnitude of the decrease of insulin receptors. As a result, the euglycemic glucose clamp technique was used to construct detailed in vivo insulin dose-response curves, including the maximum effect of insulin, for normal and obese individuals (28). Hepatic insulin resistance was found to be due to a pure decrease in insulin receptors. On the other hand, peripheral glucose disposal varied, with the least hyperinsulinemic, least insulin-resistant patients showing only a receptor defect, while the most hyperinsulinemic manifested the largest postreceptor defect. The investigators suggested "a continuous spectrum of defects as one advances from mild to severe insulin resistance" (28).

Further studies of the nature of the postreceptor defect in obesity have been carried out in human adipocytes (29) by measuring glucose transport with 3-O-methyl glucose in adipocytes from lean and obese subjects. In vitro dose-response curves were shifted to the right in obese subjects. "In those patients in whom in vivo studies showed decreased insulin sensitivity with only a rightward shift in the dose-response curve, in vitro studies also demonstrated only a rightward shift in the glucose transport dose-response curve with normal maximal responsiveness. However, in those patients who demonstrated a postreceptor defect as well as decreased insulin sensitivity in vivo similar findings were observed in vitro" (29). Thus, a strong correlation between in vivo and in vitro postreceptor defects in obesity has been shown. The nature of the defect has not yet been elucidated. As the investigators have suggested, it could be due to a decrease in the number of glucose carriers, a decrease in the affinity of the carrier for glucose, or a decrease in the accessibility of the carriers to the cell surface (29). Also, other postreceptor intracellular steps than glucose transport are likely to be involved.

DIABETES MELLITUS AND INSULIN RESISTANCE

In non-insulin-dependent Type 2 diabetes mellitus, insulin resistance occurs. In diabetic patients who are also obese, much of this resistance is due to the obesity itself. In many non-insulin-dependent diabetics, however, obesity is not present, and yet insulin resistance still occurs in most of them (30,31). There is a group of the more severe lean Type 2 diabetics, however, who do not show insulin resistance and whose basal and stimulated insulin levels are low, indicating a primary insulin deficiency rather than an insulin resistance (32). These diabetics are a minority within the Type 2 lean group; the majority, whether chemical diabetic or more severe, have generally shown normal or elevated plasma insulins (33) and a peripheral resistance to infused insulin, suggesting a target tissue insulin resistance (34,35).

Since no really satisfactory animal model of nonketotic non-insulin-dependent Type 2 diabetes occurs, the insulin resistance of the lean Type 2 diabetic has been studied directly in man in vitro utilizing human tissues and also in vivo in man. Insulin-receptor studies in such diabetics have shown decreased insulin-receptor binding to monocytes, erythrocytes, and adipocytes (36–41). The majority of studies have shown this decreased binding to be due to a decrease in the number of insulin receptors, without any change in receptor affinity (36). It is interesting that mild diabetics seem to have as decreased a receptor number as more severe diabetics (42). Thus, Olefsky and Reaven could not document a clear relation between decreased receptor number and insulin resistance (42). As mentioned, these insulin-resistant diabetics, whether they have fasting hyperglycemia or purely chemical diabetes, show a basal hyperinsulinemia associated with the decreased receptor number (43). This suggests either a down-regulation of insulin receptors by the hyperinsulinemia or a hypoinsulinemia induced secondarily by the decreased number of insulin receptors.

That there is a lack of correlation in the decrease in insulin receptors and the severity of hyperglycemia and insulin resistance in lean Type 2 diabetics suggests that defects which are beyond the insulin-binding step must be involved. In diabetic animal tissues, a defect in glucose transport in adipocytes (44) and skeletal muscle (45,46) has been found. This glucose transport abnormality has also been shown in adipocytes taken from human diabetics (47). Glucose transport is not the only abnormality occurring intracellularly. For example, glycolytic enzyme concentrations are also affected (48).

In summary, the mechanisms of insulin resistance in Type 2 diabetes are not wholly clear and are multifaceted. Decreased receptor binding seems to be primarily involved in mild glucose intolerance. In more severe disease, a combination of decreased receptor binding and postreceptor defects seems evident. These postreceptor defects may include glucose transport, enzymatic alterations, or other as yet unspecified intracellular events.

EFFECT OF DIETARY INTERVENTION ON INSULIN-RECEPTOR FUNCTION

In discussing the effect of dietary intervention on insulin sensitivity of obese and of diabetic patients, it is probably easiest to divide the diets into hypocaloric, high carbohydrate, and high fat.

Hypocaloric Diets

The most complete series of studies of the effect of hypocaloric diets on insulin binding and insulin receptors was done in ob/ob mice (17,19,21,22,49). A 24-hour period of fasting reversed receptor number toward normal and circulating insulin levels dropped. If, however, while fasting the animals, exogenous insulin was given, insulin-receptor concentration and insulin binding did not increase, suggesting that insulin itself was regulating the number of receptor sites on the cell membrane.

It is important to remember that an increase in insulin-receptor number or affinity and in insulin binding is not always associated with enhanced biological effect. Studies by Kasuga et al. (50) and Olefsky and Kobayashi (51) both showed that fasting in rats led to an increase in overall insulin binding to cells. However, glucose oxidation was markedly decreased. Thus, the increased insulin binding was not reflected in greater glucose transport or glucose oxidation, but rather the opposite.

LeMarchand et al. (52) also investigated the effect of fasting on insulin binding and on glucose metabolism in liver, muscle, and adipose tissue of ob/ob mice. They found, like Roth (1) in the same animals and like Kasuga (50) and Olefsky (51) in rats, that insulin binding was greatly increased in cells of fasted animals. This was true of all three tissues studied. However, as in the Olefsky studies, glucose oxidation was found to be decreased.

Human studies of fasting or of hypocaloric diets have also been done in obese subjects who wished to lose weight. Bar et al. (53) studied insulin-receptor function after an acute 48–72 hour fast and after a chronic diet of 600 cal/day. In the acute fast, they observed a decrease of insulin binding, which was all due to increased binding affinity, with no change in receptor number. With the chronic hypocaloric diet, which was balanced for carbohydrate, protein, and fat, plasma insulin levels were restored, insulin binding was increased, and receptor concentration returned to normal without a change in affinity. In all of the patients, the total receptor concentration was inversely related to the circulating levels of insulin measured at rest and after overnight fast. The authors concluded that "an insulin receptor undergoes in vivo modulation of its interaction with insulin by changing receptor concentration and by altering the affinity of existing receptors" (53).

Kolterman et al. (54) also studied the effect of acute and chronic starvation on insulin binding to isolated human adipocytes from obese subjects. After 72 hours of fasting there was a 38% increase in binding but no change in receptor number. These investigators, like Bar et al. (53), documented that this acute effect was due to increased receptor affinity. After a 14-day fast, there was a 150% rise in binding resulting from a further increase in receptor affinity and an increase in receptor number. Thus it is clear that the short-term hypocaloric effect is increased insulin biding due to increased affinity while the long-term effect is due to increased receptor number. The increase in receptor number is probably secondary to the decreased circulating insulin occurring with fasting for 14 days. These authors (54,55) also found that the rate at which insulin dissociates from its receptor decreased with fasting.

In anorexia nervosa, an example of hypocaloric intake taken to pathological extremes, insulin binding was found to be increased in the red blood cells due to an increase in the concentration of binding sites per cell, with little or no change in affinity. The subjects were retested after therapy for their anorexia, at a time when their weight had improved toward normal. Insulin binding and receptor number concentration decreased toward normal with weight gain.

Patients with anorexia nervosa are very sensitive to an insulin infusion (56,57), though they also tend to show abnormal glucose tolerance with sustained hyperglycemia after a glucose load (58,59). Certainly, as a group, they have lower prevailing glucose and insulin than normal weight individuals. The very sensitive response to intravenous insulin suggests exquisite tissue response to circulating insulin and the data on insulin binding referred to above are compatible with this.

High-Fat vs. High-Carbohydrate Diet

The insulin-binding effect of feeding high-fat vs. high-carbohydrate isocaloric diets to rats has been studied by Ip et al. (60). Rats were fed either of the two diets for five to ten days. The diets contained 33% of calories as protein and 67% as either lard or glucose. Isolated adipocytes from animals fed the high-fat diet showed much lower insulin binding at all levels of insulin concentration. No changes in affinity for the hormone were found. In association with this, the adipocytes of the high-fat diet rats showed a markedly decreased ^{14}C glucose oxidation. An additional inhibition of insulin action at steps beyond the receptor was suggested by the fact that spermine, which does not affect insulin binding, had a smaller insulinlike effect in these high-fat diet animals.

No difference in insulin binding and glucose oxidation was found in rats fed the high-carbohydrate diet compared to those fed normal laboratory chow (60). From this study, it could not be ascertained whether the decreased insulin binding and decreased insulin biological effect in the high-fat diet animals was caused by the high fat content or the absence of carbohydrate in the diet.

Olefsky et al. (61) also studied the effect of high-carbohydrate (fat-free) and high-fat (carbohydrate-free) diets on glucose oxidation and insulin binding in rats. The diets were similar to those used by Ip et al. (60) and the animals were given the diets for ten days. The high-carbohydrate (fat-free) diet caused a decrease in insulin binding and in the number of insulin receptors. There was also increased glucose transport and increased intracellular glucose metabolism. This would suggest increased overall cellular insulin responsiveness in the face of decreased receptors, which must be related to increased activity of steps beyond insulin binding. In contrast, the high-fat diet depressed all aspects of intracellular glucose metabolism and in conjunction with decreased receptors caused an overall insulin resistance. That high-fat feeding produces an insulin resistance had been shown previously in rats (62,63). Adipose tissue of high-fat diet rats is particularly resistant to the action of insulin on glucose metabolism (64), although muscle is also affected (63).

It is possible that the effects on receptors caused by a high-fat diet may be related to phospholipid or other changes in the plasma membrane, as suggested by Ip et al. (60). The changes seen in receptors caused by a high-carbohydrate diet may be partially related to the prevailing insulin levels, which were higher on the high-carbohydrate diet, as has been previously documented (65). As previously discussed, increased insulin levels can lead to decreased insulin binding (66).

The fact that with the high-carbohydrate diet, despite decreased insulin binding, increased glucose transport and metabolism occur, suggests that the chronic prevailing high insulin effect on the cells is crucial. That the effect of insulin is key in setting the cellular glucose transport and metabolism activity is supported by the lower glucose oxidative capacity of adipocytes taken from rats in hypoinsulinemic states, such as fasting (67) or streptozotocin diabetes (68), while glucose oxidative capacity is increased in rats made hyperinsulinemic (69).

The effect of high-carbohydrate diet has also been tested in man. Previous studies of high-carbohydrate diets in mild diabetes had reported increased insulin sensitivity and enhanced glucose tolerance (70,71). In contrast, Horton (72) showed that high-fat, low-carbohydrate diets impaired the responsiveness of glucose uptake to insulin of both adipose tissue and muscle in man. Salans et al. (73) showed that when carbohydrate was isocalorically substituted for fat in the diet, insulin responsiveness of isolated fat cells, as measured by glucose oxidation and glyceride-glycerol synthesis, was increased. Kolterman et al. (74) studied the effects of short-term (five days) and long-term (two weeks) high-carbohydrate diets on insulin binding to isolated adipocytes and insulin sensitivity in vivo in normal subjects. The diets compared were 43% carbohydrate, 42% fat, and 15% protein vs. 75% carbohydrate, 10% fat, 15% protein. Insulin sensitivity was measured by the infusion of a combination of insulin, glucose, epinephrine, and propranolol, with which suppression of endogenous insulin secretion occurs and steady-state plasma concentrations of glucose and insulin are achieved. Comparable steady-state plamsa levels of exogenous insulin are achieved in each subject and thus the ability of different groups of subjects to dispose of comparable glucose loads can be measured (74).

The high-carbohydrate diet caused hyperinsulinemia throughout the day in both the short-term and long-term diet groups. This was associated with decreased insulin binding to isolated adipocytes. In the short-term group the decreased binding was due to decreased insulin affinity in the adipocytes, while in the long-term group it was due to an actual decrease in receptor number. Despite this decrease in binding, however, total in vivo insulin sensitivity was markedly improved in both the short- and long-term groups.

Thus, as previously described in rats (60,61), human subjects on a high-carbohydrate diet paradoxically have enhanced insulin sensitivity despite decreased binding affinity and/or receptor number. This must be due to an alteration of steps beyond the insulin receptor, leading to improved glucose transport and glucose metabolism.

SULFONYLUREAS AND RECEPTOR FUNCTION

The introduction of oral drugs with hypoglycemic action was received with enthusiasm by both doctors and their diabetic patients who were unhappy with injectable insulin. The acceptability of the oral sulfonylurea agents, five of which are presently being marketed in this country, has been greatly marred by the University Group Diabetes Study, which implicated at least one of them (tolbutamide) in an increased incidence of cardiac deaths (75). Without delving into that controversy, however, there is little doubt about the hypoglycemic efficacy of these drugs, and it is the mechanism of this glucose-lowering effect which will be discussed here.

The sulfonylureas stimulate insulin release from the islets of Langerhans. This occurs in man, experimental animals, in vitro preparations of perfused pancreas, and isolated islets (76). Clinical studies soon showed, however, that whereas early in treatment with a sulfonylurea such as chlorpropamide, postmeal insulin rose and glucose fell, after long-term therapy (over five weeks), the glucose remained low while the elevated insulin dropped once more to original low levels (77). This loss of insulin elevation with a sustained hypoglycemia effect was confirmed by a number of investigators with a number of different sulfonylurea preparations (78–81).

The puzzling observation of sustained hypoglycemia despite a normalization downwards of the insulin levels raised speculation that extrapancreatic effects of the sulfonylurea agents might occur with chronic therapy (80,82). Searle et al. (83) showed an increase in ^{14}C-glucose utilization in normal subjects given tolbutamide, though they could not show this in diabetics. Blumenthal (84) documented a potentiating effect in vitro of chlorpropamide on the hepatic action of insulin, showing that glucagon-stimulated glucose production by the liver could be inhibited.

Feldman and Lebovitz (80), using chronic glybenclamide therapy for two to six months, reported a continuous improvement of glucose tolerance with decreasing insulin levels, and suggested that the decreasing insulin-to-glucose ratios implied an extrapancreatic mechanism of action. Duckworth et al. (81) chronically administered glyburide to a group of previously untreated nonketotic diabetics. Glucose tolerance was significantly improved in these diabetics over pretreatment values after six months of treatment even though insulin levels were not raised over control values. The investigators asserted that the effect of sulfonylureas on insulin secretion did not completely explain the action of the sulfonylureas, and suggested that an extrapancreatic effect of glyburide was likely. Similar studies subsequently were reported for other sulfonylurea drugs, such as tolbutamide (79), tolazamide (85), and chloropropamide (86).

Lebovitz et al. (87,88) assessed insulin action by measuring insulin-mediated glucose disposal in nonketotic diabetic patients after glipizide therapy. The glucose disposal of these patients was increased while they took the glipizide, suggesting that the drug potentiated insulin action and ameliorated insulin resistance.

Greenfield et al. (89) also studied the effect of glipizide treatment on diabetic control and on in vivo insulin secretion and action in patients with non-insulin-dependent diabetes mellitus. An insulin-clamp technique was used whereby a continuous infusion of insulin was given and the amount of glucose disposal was calculated by also infusing glucose to maintain a constant level in the blood. Increased glucose disposal, that is, greater insulin sensitvity, occurred after three months of glipizide therapy. Also, insulin suppression tests were done with an infusion of epinephrine, propanolol, glucose, and insulin. As mentioned previously, under these conditions endogenous insulin secretion is inhibited and glucose uptake is stimulated by the infused exogenous insulin. The level of steady-state glucose reached after a given time is a measure of insulin sensitivity. This again was improved after glipizide therapy. Thus, chronic therapy with glipizide led to an increased in vivo insulin action.

These results are compatible with a substantial extrapancreatic effect of the sulfonylurea on insulin action.

Best et al. (90) studied patients with untreated non-insulin-dependent diabetes before and after therapy with chlorpropamide for three to six months. During therapy, fasting plasma glucose and glucose production rate were lower. Fasting plasma insulin increased in some but not all patients. When a low-dose insulin infusion was given to approximate the increases of portal venous insulin during therapy, similar falls of glucose production occurred. The authors concluded that inhibition of endogenous glucose production during chronic chlorpropamide therapy lowers fasting glucose and that enhanced insulin secretion is an important mechanism for this. However, since the effect was observed even in patients with no detectable rise in plasma insulin, an additional contribution by some other extrapancreatic mechanism seemed likely.

EFFECT OF SULFONYLUREAS ON INSULIN BINDING

As mentioned previously, insulin-receptor studies have shown that Type 2 diabetic patients have insulin resistance of variable severity and as the severity increases, insulin-receptor number drops (91). Olefsky and Reaven (91) treated a group of such insulin-resistant nonobese diabetic patients for one to three months with chlorpropamide. This therapy was associated with a significant increase in monocyte insulin receptors in 13 of the 16 subjects studied. No decrease in insulin affinity of the target cells was found. These results clearly demonstrated that mononuclear leukocytes isolated from adult nonketotic, nonobese diabetics with fasting hyperglycemia have a decreased ability to bind insulin and that the binding capacity was improved with sulfonylurea therapy (91).

Feinglos and Lebovitz (92) tried to clarify the extrapancreatic mechanism of sulfonylurea action by examining the insulin sensitivity of mice given glipizide. These treated animals developed increased insulin sensitivity in comparison to controls. The insulin binding to purified liver plasma membranes was then studied. Scatchard plots of insulin binding by these purified hepatic plasma membranes showed similarly shaped curves, indicating that glipizide did not alter affinity to insulin. In contrast, however, the liver membranes of the glipizide-treated mice bound twice as much insulin as those of the controls. Thus, the potentiation of insulin action on glucose disposal (87) was consistent with a glipizide-induced increase in the number of available insulin receptors on the plasma membranes of responsive tissues. The mechanism by which the sulfonylureas induced increased receptor number was unclear.

A subsequent study by Beck-Nielsen et al. (93) examined the effect of glibenclamide on the insulin receptors, insulin sensitivity, and insulin secretion of obese, nonketotic Type 2 diabetics. The diabetics were studied before and after ten days' treatment with a 1200 kcal diet or a 1200 kcal diet plus 10 mg of glibenclamide. In the group treated with diet alone, no change in insulin secretory pattern was found, but insulin sensitivity improved by 37% and insulin binding to monocytes increased owing to a 36% increase in binding affinity. In the group treated with glibenclamide and diet the insulin secretory pattern was unchanged, but the insulin sensitivity increased 83%. Insulin binding was increased owing to an 80% rise in the number of insulin receptors.

Recently, Archer (94) has reported on insulin receptors in nonobese, nonketotic Type 2 diabetics whom she treated first for two weeks with tolbutamide and then after an interim two-week "washout" period, for two weeks with tolazamide. She compared the insulin binding to erythrocytes from normal lean subjects with the binding to erythrocytes from the sulfonylurea-treated subjects. Erythrocytes from normal individuals bound twice as much insulin as those of diabetics. Scatchard analysis showed that the cells of normal subjects had approximately twice the number of receptor sites as those of diabetic subjects.

The postsulfonylurea therapy insulin-binding studies showed no change in binding after two weeks of tolbutamide, but a definite increase in binding and in receptor site number after two weeks of tolazamide. Further studies in volunteer diabetics were then done with 90 days of tolazamide treatment. Insulin binding was increased by about 25%. These changes in insulin receptors occurred without change in body weight. This study suggests that different sulfonylurea drugs may have different effects on receptor concentration. However, this negative report with tolbutamide must be balanced with a positive report (95) which did find increased insulin binding with tolbutamide therapy in Type 2 diabetics.

Prince and Olefsky recently investigated the effect of glyburide in vitro on cultured human fibroblasts. Sulfonylurea increased receptor number and also partially inhibited the usual down-regulation of insulin receptors induced by insulin in these cultured fibroblasts (96). This suggests that the sulfonylurea-induced change in insulin-receptor number is a direct effect and not mediated via a change in circulating insulin level. These investigators suggested that the sulfonylurea increased insulin binding by inhibiting the internalization of the hormone-bound receptor.

POSTRECEPTOR ACTION OF SULFONYLUREAS

In the studies discussed above on the increase in insulin binding and in-sulin receptors induced by chronic sulfonylurea therapy, the effect of these binding changes on insulin sensitivity was generally not investi-gated because the studies were done on plasma membrane fractions (92) or cells not responsive to insulin (46,48,93). It is very difficult to sort out the direct effects of the sulfonylurea drugs on target tissues since as the diabetic state improves many substrate and hormonal changes accom-pany this improvement. Because of this, Maloff and Lockwood (97) have utilized adipose tissue in a long-term incubation system. In such a system direct effects of the drug, unobfuscated by other concurrent in vivo changes of drug therapy, might be identified more easily.

Rat adipose tissue was incubated for 20 to 44 hours in the presence or absence of tolazamide. Insulin-receptor number and insulin-receptor af-finity were measured with and without the drug and no change could be found with drug treatment. Glucose uptake as measured by either 2-deoxyglucose or 3-O-methylglucose transport was not increased in the absence of insulin. However, with tolazamide in the incubation medium there was a potentiation of insulin action on glucose transport of about 30% at all insulin concentrations tested from 0.4 to 40 ng/ml. Conversion of glucose to CO_2 and total lipids was also increased. These studies on rat adipocytes suggest an effect of tolazamide not on the insulin receptor but rather on postreceptor insulin action, particularly on insulin-mediated glucose transport into the cell.

Because their data do not support the hypothesis that the primary extrapancreatic action of the sulfonylureas is to increase receptor num-ber, Maloff and Lockwood have proposed that "the enhanced insulin binding seen with long-term administration of sulfonylureas may be a function of the concurrent decrease in plasma insulin levels rather than a primary effect of the drugs" (97). Certainly, it is well-known that insu-lin receptors can be regulated directly by insulin itself (98,99). Since many non-insulin-dependent diabetics have high insulin levels, these high insulin levels could down-regulate the receptors, whose numbers could rise again as insulin fell with sulfonylurea treatment.

In conclusion, it is likely that the sulfonylurea action on peripheral tissues, like the dietary one, is a combination of effect on insulin recep-tors and on postreceptor function. It is clear, however, that an extrapancreatic effect is present and must be considered important in the overall therapeutic effectiveness of the sulfonylurea drugs in diabe-tes mellitus.

REFERENCES

1. R. S. Bar, L. C. Harrison, M. Muggeo, P. Gorden, C. R. Kahn, and J. Roth, *Advances Intern. Med.*, **24**, 23 (1979).

2. C. R. Kahn and J. Roth, in G. S. Levey, Ed., *Hormone-Receptor Interaction: Molecular Aspects*, Marcel Dekker, N.Y., 1976.

3. C. R. Kahn, D. M. Neville, Jr., and J. Roth, *J. Biol. Chem.*, **248**, 244 (1973).

4. J. R. Gavin, III, J. Roth, D. M. Neville, P. DeMeyts, and D. N. Buell, *Proc. Natl. Acad Sci, U.S.A.*, **71**, 84 (1974).

5. D. Rabinowitz and K. L. Zierler, *J. Clin. Invest.*, **41**, 2173 (1962).

6. J. M. Olefsky, G. M. Reaven, and J. W. Farquhar, *J. Clin. Invest.*, **53**, 64 (1974).

7. R. A. Kreisberg, B. R. Boshell, J. DiPlacido, and R. J. Roddman, *New Engl. J. Med.*, **276**, 314 (1967).

8. J. M. Olefsky, in *Current Concepts*, Upjohn and Co., 1980.

9. R. C. Kahn, *Metabolism*, **27**, 1893 (1978).

10. T. Kono and F. W. Barham, *J. Biol. Chem.*, **246**, 6210 (1971).

11. R. S. Bar, C. R. Kahn, and H. S. Koren, *Nature*, **265**, 632 (1977).

12. R. J. Muschel, N. Rosen, O. M. Rosen, and B. R. Bloom, *J. Immunol.*, **119**, 1813 (1977).

13. J. A. Archer, P. Gorden, and J. Roth, *J. Clin. Invest.*, **55**, 166 (1975).

14. J. M. Olefsky, *J. Clin. Invest.*, **57**, 1165 (1976).

15. J. Roth, C. R. Kahn, M. A. Lesniak, P. Gorden, P. DeMeyts, K. Megyesi, D. M. Neville, Jr., J. R. Gavin, III, A. H. Soll, P. Freychet, I. D. Goldfine, R. S. Bar, and J. A. Archer, *Recent Prog. Horm. Res.*, **31**, 95 (1976).

16. O. G. Kolterman, G. M. Reaven, and J. M. Olefsky, *J. Clin. Endocrinol. Metab.*, **48**, 487 (1976).

17. P. Freychet, M. H. Laudat, P. Laudat, G. Rosselin, C. R. Kahn, P. Gorden, and J. Roth, *F.E.B.S. Lett.*, **25**, 339 (1972).

18. A. H. Soll, C. R. Kahn, and D. M. Neville, Jr., *J. Biol. Chem.*, **250**, 7402, 1975.

19. A. H. Soll, C. R. Kahn, D. M. Neville, Jr., and J. Roth, *J. Clin. Invest.*, **56**, 769 (1975).

20. J. M. Olefsky, *J. Clin. Invest.*, **57**, 842 (1976).

21. A. H. Soll, I. D. Goldfine, J. Roth, R. Kahn, and D. M. Neville, *J. Biol. Chem.*, **249**, 4127 (1974).

22. A. H. Soll, C. R. Kahn, and D. M. Neville, Jr., *J. Biol. Chem.*, **250**, 7402 (1975).

23. J. N. Livingston and D. H. Lockwood, *Biochem. Biophys. Res. Commun.*, **61**, 989 (1974).

24. M. O. Czech, *J. Clin. Invest.*, **57**, 1523 (1976).

25. M. DiGirolamo and D. Rudman, *Endocrinol.*, **82**, 1133 (1968).

26. L. B. Salans and J. W. Dougherty, *J. Clin. Invest.*, **50**, 1399 (1971).

27. Y. Le-Marchand-Brustel, B. Jeanrenaud, and P. Freychet, *Am. J. Physiol.*, **234**, E348 (1978).

28. O. G. Kolterman, J. Insel, M. Saekow, and J. M. Olefsky, *J. Clin. Invest.*, **65**, 1272 (1980).

29. T. P. Giaraldi, O. C. Kolterman, and J. M. Olefsky, *J. Clin. Invest.*, **68**, 875 (1981).

30. G. M. Reaven, R. Bernstein, B. Davis, and J. M. Olefsky, *Am. J. Med.*, **60**, 80 (1976).

31. J. M. Olefsky, *Diabetes*, **25**, 1154 (1976).

32. R. A. Rizza, L. J. Mandarino, and J. E. Gerich, *Diabetes*, **30**, 990 (1981).

33. R. Chiles and M. Tzagournis, *Diabetes*, **19**, 458 (1970).

34. F. P. Alford, F. J. R. Martin, and M. J. Pearson, *Diabetologia*, **7**, 173 (1971).

35. J. M. Olefsky, M. Sperling, and G. M. Reaven, *Diabetologia*, **13**, 327 (1977).

36. J. M. Olefsky and G. M. Reaven, *J. Clin. Invest.* **54**, 1323 (1974).

37. J. M. Olefsky and G. M. Reaven, *J. Clin. Endocrinol. Metab.*, **43**, 226 (1976).

38. G. Lenti, B. Pagano, and M. Cassader, *Journees Annuelles de Diabetologie de l'Hotel Dieu*, Flammarion, Paris, 1978, p. 73.

39. P. Pagano, M. Cassader, M. Messobrio, C. Bozzo, G. Trossanelli, G. Menato, and G. Lenti, *Horm. Metab. Res.*, **12**, 177 (1980).

40. T. Robinson, J. Archer, K. Gambhir, V. Hollis, L. Carter, and C. Bradley, *Science*, **205**, 200 (1979).

41. R. DePirro, A. Fusco, R. Lauro, I. Testa, F. Ferreti, and C. DeMartins, *Diabetes*, **29**, 96 (1980).

42. J. M. Olefsky and G. M. Reaven, *Diabetes*, **26**, 680 (1977).

43. J. M. Olefsky and G. M. Reaven, *Am. J. Med.*, **60**, 89 (1976).

44. M. Kobayashi and J. M. Olefsky, *J. Clin. Invest.*, **62**, 73 (1978).

45. D. M. Kipnis and D. F. Cori, *J. Biol. Chem.*, **234**, 171 (1959).

46. H. E. Morgan, M. S. Henderson, D. M. Regen, and C. R. Park, *Ann. N.Y. Acad. Sci.*, **82**, 387 (1959).

47. D. J. Galton and J. P. D. Wilson, *Clin. Sci.*, **38**, 661 (1970).

48. D. J. Galton and J. P. D. Wilson, *Clin. Sci.*, **41**, 545 (1971).

49. M. E. Forgue and P. Freychet, *Diabetes*, **24**, 715 (1975).

50. M. Kasuga, Y. Akanuma, Y. Iwamoto, and K. Kosaka, *Endocrinol.*, **100**, 1384 (1977).

51. J. M. Olefsky and M. Kobayashi, *J. Clin. Invest.*, **61**, 329 (1978).

52. Y. LeMarchand, E. G. Loten, F. Assimocopoulos-Jeannet, M. E. Forgue, P. Freychet, and B. Jeanrenaud, *Diabetes*, **26**, 582 (1977).

53. R. S. Bar, P. Gordon, J. Roth, C. R. Kahn, and P. DeMeyts, *J. Clin. Invest.*, **58**, 1123 (1976).

54. O. G. Kolterman, M. Saekow, and J. M. Olefsky, *J. Clin. Endocr. Metab.*, **48**, 836 (1979).

55. H. Wachs013ght-Rodbard, H. A. Gross, D. Rodbard, M. H. Ebert, and J. Roth, *N. Engl. J. Med.*, **300**, 882 (1979).

56. J. Landon, F. C. Greenwood, T. C. B. Stamp, and V. Wynn, *J. Clin. Invest.*, **45**, 437 (1966).

57. J. G. Devlin, *J. Ir. Med. Assoc.*, **68**, 227 (1975).

58. E. D. Bartels, *Acta. Med. Scand.*, **124**, 185 (1946).

59. J. A. Kanis, P. Brown, K. Fitzpatrick, et al., *Q.J. Med.*, **43**, 321 (1974).

60. C. Ip, H. M. Tepperman, P. Holohan, and J. Tepperman, *J. Lipid Res.*, **17**, 588 (1976).

61. J. M. Olefsky and M. Saekow, *Endocrinol.*, **103**, 2252 (1978).

62. N. Zaragoza-Hermans and J. P. Felber, *Horm. Metab. Res.*, **4**, 25 (1972).

63. C. Susini and M. Lavau, *Diabetes*, **27**, 114 (1978).

64. M. Lavau, M. Nadeau, and C. Susini, *Biochimie*, **54**, 1057 (1972).

65. W. Grey and D. Kipnis, *N. Engl. J. Med.*, **285**, 827 (1971).

66. J. R. Gavin, III, J. Roth, D. M. Neville, Jr., P. DeMeyts, and D. N. Buell, *Proc. Natl. Acad. Sci.*, **71**, 84 (1974).

67. J. M. Olefsky, *J. Clin. Invest.*, **58**, 1450 (1976).

68. M. Kasgua, Y. Akanuma, Y. Iwamoto, and K. Kosaka, *Am. J. Physiol.*, **232**, E175, 1978.

69. M. Kobayashi and J. M. Olefsky, *Diabetologia*, **17**, 111, 1979.

70. H. P. Himsworth, *Clin. Sci.*, **1**, 1 (1933).

71. J. D. Brunzell, R. L. Lerner, W. R. Hazzard, D. Porte, Jr., and E. L. Bierman, *N. Engl. J. Med.*, **284**, 521, 1971.

72. E. S. Horton, E. Danforth, Jr., E. A. H. Sims, and L. B. Salans, *D.H.E.W. Publ. No. (NIH) 75-708, 1975, p. 323.*

73. L. B. Salans, G. A. Bray, S. W. Cushman, E. Danforth, Jr., J. A. Glennon, E. S. Horton, and E. A. H. Sims, *J. Clin. Invest.*, **53**, 848 (1974).

74. O. G. Kolterman, M. Greenfield, G. M. Reaven, M. Saeko, and J. M. Olefsky, *Diabetes*, **28**, 731 (1979).

75. University Group Diabetes Program, "A Study of the Effects of Hypoglycemic Agents on Vascular Complications in Patients with Adult-Onset Diabetes. II. Mortality Results." *Diabetes*, **19** (Suppl), 789 (1970).

76. A. Widstrom and E. Cerasi, *Acta Endocrinol.*, **72**, 506 (1973).

77. P. C. Chu, M. J. Conway, H. A. Krouse, and C. J. Goodner, *Ann. Intern. Med.*, **68**, 757 (1968).

78. A. J. Barnes, M. F. Crowley, K. J. T. Garbien, and A. Bloom, *Lancet* **2** (1974).

79. B. R. Boshell, O. J. Fox, R. F. Roddam, *et al.* in W. J. H. Butterfield, and W. Van Westering, Eds., *Tolbutamide After Ten Years*, Internat'l Congress Series No. 149, Excerpta Medica, Amsterdam, 1967, p. 286.

80. J. M. Feldman and H. E. Lebovitz, *Diabetes*, **20**, 745 (1971).

81. W. C. Duckworth, S. S. Solomon, and A. E. Kitabchi, *J. Clin. Endocrinol. Metab.*, **35**, 585 (1972).

82. J. M. Feldman and H. E. Lebovitz, *Diabetes*, **18**, 529 (1969).

83. G. L. Searle, G. E. Mortimore, R. E. Buckley, and W. A. Reilly, *Diabetes*, **8**, 167 (1959).

84. S. A. Blumenthal, *Diabetes*, **26**, 485 (1977).

85. J. R. Turtle, *Br. Med. J.*, **2**, 606 (1970).

86. G. Reaven and J. Dray, *Diabetes*, **16**, 487 (1967).

87. H. E. Lebovitz, M. N. Feinglos, H. K. Bucholtz, and F. L. Lebovitz, *J. Clin. Endocrinol. Metab.*, **45**, 601 (1977).

88. H. Lebovitz and M. N. Feinglos, *Adv. Exptl. Med. Biol.*, **119**, 371 (1979).

89. M. S. Greenfield, L. Doberne, M. Rosenthal, B. Schulz, A. Widstrom, and G. M. Reaven, *Diabetes*, **31**, 307 (1982).

90. J. D. Best, R. G. Judzewitsch, M. A. Pfeifer, J. C. Beard, J. B. Halter, and D. Porte, Jr., *Diabetes*, **31**, 333 (1982).

91.   J. M. Olefsky and G. M. Reaven, *J. Clin. Invest.*, **54,** 1323 (1974).

92.   M. N. Feinglos and H. E. Lebovitz, *Nature*, **276,** 184 (1978).

93.   H. Beck-Nielsen, H. Pedersen, and H. O. Lindskov, *Acta Endocrinol.*, **90,** 451 (1979).

94.   J. A. Archer, Tolinase Symposium Paper, Upjohn and Co., May, 1979.

95.   J. M. Olefsky and G. M. Reaven, *Am. J. Med.*, **60,** 89 (1976).

96.   M. J. Prince and J. M. Olfesky, *J. Clin. Invest.*, **66,** 608 (1980).

97.   B. L. Maloff and D. H. Lockwood, *J. Clin. Invest.*, **68,** 85 (1981).

98.   J. N. Livingston, B. J. Purvis, and D. H. Lockwood, *Metab. Clin. Exp.*, **27,** 2009 (1978).

99.   J. M. Olefsky and G. M. Reaven, *Diabetes*, **26,** 680 (1977).

9

Drugs and Nutrient Absorption

DAPHNE A. ROE, M.D.

Cornell University, Ithaca, New York

Knowledge of nutritional physiology and biochemistry as well as pharmacology has inclined us to the view that it is possible to differentiate drugs from nutrients with respect to chemistry, absorption, metabolism, elimination, function, and toxicity. Such rigorous differentiations of drugs and nutrients is no longer possible because nutrients in pharmacological doses behave as drugs, and food or beverage sources of nutrients may contain natural substances or additives which behave as foreign compounds or drugs. Thus, while it is still possible to define a nutrient and a drug and in the present context to compare and contrast the modes of absorption of these two classes of compounds, the overlap must not be overlooked. Indeed, when answering the question of which drugs significantly affect nutrient absorption, or the companion question, when do drugs significantly affect nutrient absorption, it is important to include nutrients as drugs, and nonnutrient energy sources as well as nonnutrient, noncaloric dietary substances as pharmacological agents.

OVERVIEW OF DRUGS AND NUTRIENTS WITH UPDATE ON THEIR ABSORPTION

Drugs and Drug Absorption

Drugs have been defined as chemical agents other than food which affect living organisms (1). In the medicinal sense, however, a drug is any chemical agent used in the diagnosis, prevention, or treatment of disease. Perhaps we should add that drugs, also in the medicinal sense, are

129

compounds used to alter mood, to prevent pregnancy, or to affect destiny. Alternatively, we can adopt the biochemical definition of a drug as being any compound that affects the living organisms and that does not enter into *normal* biosynthetic pathways within the body. With all the limitations of these definitions, it seems clear that most drugs are treated by the body as foreign compounds, that few drugs nourish the body, and that a relatively few drugs are utilized by the body for maintenance of physiological function.

Drug absorption, in the present context, pertains to uptake after oral administration. Absorption of drugs may be divided into an intraluminal phase and a mucosal phase. The intraluminal phase can be described as preparative.

Solid drug preparations undergo dissolution in the gastrointestinal contents and it is necessary that the drug be dissolved before it can traverse the gastrointestinal mucosa. Several mechanisms of gastrointestinal drug absorption have been described both for lipid-soluble and for polar compounds. Lipid-soluble drugs readily undergo passive absorption and penetrate the intestinal epithelium through the lipoprotein barrier. Transport of small molecular weight water-soluble drugs may be through aqueous pores in the intestinal mucosa, which have an average radius in the proximal jejunum of 7.5 Å and in the ileum of 3.5 Å.

The transfer of most drugs, whether by direct membrane transport (the major route) or through aqueous pore (the minor route), is by passive diffusion. The nonionized form of acidic and basic drugs is preferentially absorbed. Both the dissociation constant of the drug and the pH of the gastrointestinal environment define the fraction of the drug that is ionized. The dissociation constant is expressed as pKa, which is the negative logarithm of the acidic dissociation constant.

Carrier-mediated transport or active transport of drugs is uncommon except when the drug is a structural analog of a natural compound (2). Factors affecting drug absorption are listed in Table 1. Although orally administered drugs can be absorbed in the mouth, esophagus, stomach, duodenum, jejunum, ileum, colon, or rectum, drug absorption is mainly within the small intestine because of the enormous surface area offered by the villi and microvilli.

Nutrients and Nutrient Absorption

Nutrients are naturally occurring elements and compounds of plants or animal origin that may be ingested in food and water or synthesized within or outside the body. They are required for growth as well as for

Table 1. Physical, Chemical, and Physiological Factors Affecting Drug Absorption

1. Drug characteristics

    Lipid solubility
    pKa
    Drug form (solid/liquid)
    Particle size
    Particle conformation and surface area
    Coating
    Additives

2. Gastrointestinal tract characteristics

    A. Mucosal
    Epithelial form
    Epithelial integrity
    Surface area
    pH at brush border
    Intestinal mucosal metabolism

    B. Vascular
    Splanchnic blood flow

    C. Motility
    Gastric emptying time
    Intestinal transit time

    D. Intraluminal
    Precipitation
    Adsorption
    Ion exchange
    Complexation

the structural and functional integrity of all living organisms. However, in pharmacological doses nutrients have other defined functions including photoprotection (β carotene), vasodilatation (niacin), hypocholesterolemic effect (niacin), prevention of organic brain damage (thiamin in Wernicke's encephalopathy), and prevention of oxidative damage (vitamin E). Nutrients present in food require gastric, pancreatic, and intestinal digestion before absorption. Descriptions of nutrient digestion and absorption are to be found in standard texts of physiology and nutrition (3–5).

Nutrient absorption is by active and carrier-mediated transport, by passive diffusion, and by pinocytosis. In humans, after the perinatal period, absorption of physiological loads of nutrients is largely by active or energy-requiring processes. An extensive update on nutrient absorption was published in 1980(6), and in the last two years, there have also been several major reviews of vitamin absorption. Rose (7) prefaced his description of the absorption of water-soluble vitamins by the statement "The reader familiar with textbook accounts of vitamin absorption may be surprised to find that evidence now exists in favor of a specialized transport mechanism for nearly all vitamins. . . ." However, readers of Rose's review should be aware that whereas active transport of water-soluble vitamins is stressed, such mechanisms are most important when physiological doses of these vitamins are ingested in foods or in synthetic foods.

ABSORPTION OF PHARMACOLOGICAL VERSUS PHYSIOLOGICAL DOSES OF WATER-SOLUBLE VITAMINS

Folic Acid and the Folacins

In human subjects absorption of certain water-soluble vitamins, for example folacins, is different when the vitamin is ingested in pharmacological as contrasted with physiological amounts. Further, the metabolism or interconversion of folacins during absorption depends on the folacin vitamer ingested. Deconjugation of folacin polyglutamates occurs during absorption, and this enzymatic hydrolysis is by the intracellular carboxypeptidase folate (folacin) conjugase (8).

Nonmethylated dietary folacins at physiological levels may be converted to 5-methyl-tetrahydrofolate (MTHF) in the jejunal mucosa and the 5-MTHF is then absorbed. In the rat, absorption of 5-MTHF is by a nonsaturable transport mechanism, probably simple diffusion, but in the human, there is a saturable and specialized transport process for folacins (9,10).

Absorption of pharmacological doses of folic acid is different from absorption of physiological levels of the vitamin. Chapman et al. (11), using high pressure liquid chromatography (HPLC) techniques, found that when normal human subjects received 0.169 mg/kg of folic acid by mouth, four hours later the serum contained more folacin as folic acid than as 5-MTHF.

We have recently confirmed these observations on folacin absorption and we predict that with HPLC it will very soon be possible to describe the effects of food and drug variables not only on the level of folacin absorption, but also on the forms of folacin absorbed.

Riboflavin

Absorption of pharmacological doses of riboflavin and of riboflavin-5'-phosphate has been extensively studied in human subjects. Most of the human studies have employed the riboflavin load test, in which subjects are first saturated with riboflavin. Urinary riboflavin is estimated for the 24 hours before the test and on the test day each subject receives a pharmacological dose of riboflavin or FMN by mouth. Thereafter, fractioned urine samples are collected for post-load estimation of riboflavin. The assumption is made that the greater the concentration of riboflavin in sequential post-load urines, the greater the absorption of the vitamin, and the sooner after the load that riboflavin concentration peaks in the urine, the more rapid the absorption of the vitamin.

With this test, a number of factors have been identified which influence riboflavin absorption. Studies have compared absorption of riboflavin and FMN, and FMN absorption is faster because it is more soluble within the gastrointestinal tract. Dietary factors that "promote" riboflavin absorption, as reflected by this change in the load tests, include ingestion of food, intake of dietary fiber, particularly coarse bran, intake of cola beverages, and a glucose polymer used as a caloric supplement (12–14). Drugs that promote riboflavin absorption include anticholinergics. Conditions that increase absorption of riboflavin can be divided into those which increase vitamin solubilization and those which slow gastric emptying time and optimize the rate at which riboflavin is delivered to the absorption site in the proximal part of the small intestine.

The precise mechanism whereby riboflavin is absorbed is still unsettled. However, it is known that the phosphorylated form of the vitamin in food is rapidly dephosphorylated in the intestinal lumen, and this finding has suggested that the free form of the vitamin is absorbed (12).

Table 2.   Factors Influencing the Absorption of Pharmacological Doses of Folic Acid and Riboflavin

Vitamin	Folic Acid	Riboflavin
Pharmaceutical factors	Dose Dosage form	Form Dose Dosage form
Dietary factors	Glucose or glucose polymer intake ↑	Food ↑ Fiber ↑ Cola beverages ↑ Glucose polymer ↑
Drugs	Folacin antagonists ↓ Anion exchange resins ↓ Antacids ↓	Anticholinergics ↑ Thyroxine ↓ Cathartics ↓

When the vitamin enters the intestinal mucosal cells, it undergoes rephosphorylation (15).

The more we learn about the absorption of pharmacological doses of the vitamins folic acid and riboflavin, the more we come to realize that when the dose of these nutrients is high, absorption is influenced by factors that are more analogous to factors which promote or retard drug absorption than to physiological factors. Information on major variables that alter absorption of large doses of folic acid and riboflavin is summarized in Table 2.

DRUG-INDUCED MALABSORPTION OF NUTRIENTS

Drug-induced malabsorption can be due to intraluminal events, drug toxicity, or drug events occurring outside the gastrointestinal tract (Table 3).

Table 3. Classification of Drug-Induced Malabsorption

Mechanism	Drug Causing
A. Intraluminal	
Solubilization	Mineral oil
Chelation	Tetracycline
Formation of insoluble product	Aluminum and magnesium hydroxide
Adsorption and complexation	Cholestyramine Colestipol
Maldigestion	
Gastric	Cimetidine
Pancreatic[a]	Ethanol
Intestinal	Neomycin
Biliary[a]	Cholestyramine
B. Mucosal	
↑ Brush border pH	Antacids
Loss of structural integrity	Colchicine, MTX
Loss of binding site	PAS
↓ Active transport	Diphenylhydantoin

[a]See discussion of nonenterogeneous malabsorption in text.

Intraluminal Events

Intraluminal events leading to nutrient malabsorption include solubilization of a nutrient in the drug, adsorption of the nutrient onto the drug, which may be nonspecific or by ion exchange, precipitation of the nutrient by the drug to form an insoluble product, or change in pH with or without drug-induced maldigestion. Drug-induced reduction in intestinal transit time cannot so cause malabsorption.

The solution of beta carotene in mineral oil renders this vitamin unavailable (16). Adsorption of folic acid onto the anion-exchange resin cholestyramine reduces absorption (17). Intake of massive amounts of the antacids magnesium and aluminum hydroxide causes precipitation of dietary phosphate. With chronic excessive use of antacids, this leads to phosphorus depletion and secondary osteomalacia (18,19). Antacids can also increase the pH at the brush border of the proximal small intestine and so reduce folacin absorption (20).

Uptake of vitamin B_{12} in the ileum is also dependent on the pH of the environment. Absorption is maximal at pH 6.6 and above and absent below pH 5.5. Reduced absorption of vitamin B_{12} has been found with intake of slow-release preparations of potassium chloride (21,22). Because it reduces gastric acid secretion and pepsin release, cimetidine diminishes gastric digestion and the release of vitamin B_{12} from animal protein food. The availability of vitamin B_{12} for combination with gastric intrinsic factor is thereby reduced, which can impair absorption (23).

Laxatives and cathartics can cause malabsorption in part because of excessively rapid passage of gut contents through the small intestine. It is very questionable whether this effect of laxatives or cathartics on gut motility is ever the sole cause of malabsorption associated with laxative abuse. Rather, laxative-induced malabsorption is due to an increase in gut motility plus mucosal change induced by specific drugs such as phenolphthalein, bisacodyl, or senna (24–26).

Mucosal Toxicity

Alcohol is a drug which, when it is abused, is highly toxic to the intestinal mucosa. In men and women who are alcoholics, spree drinking can cause an acute and reversible malabsorption syndrome. Alcohol has been shown to inhibit active transport and absorption of nutrients including amino acids (27), electrolytes (28), long-chain fatty acids (29), thiamin (30), and folacin (31). Structural changes in the gut mucosa in spree drinking alcoholics include megaloblastosis due to folacin deficiency (32). Brush border structure and enzyme function are also impaired, causing a high prevalence of lactose intolerance in actively drinking alcoholics (33).

In Crohn's disease, patients' folacin malabsorption may be due to administration of sulfasalazine (Azulfidine). This drug is a folacin antagonist and it impairs folacin transport across the intestinal epithelium. However, folacin deficiency in patients with this disease is the outcome of the drug therapy, of malabsorption due to the inflammatory bowel disease, and of low dietary folacin (34).

Selective drug-induced nutrient malabsorption is well documented. Thus the biguanide metformin has been reported to cause vitamin B_{12} malabsorption with megaloblastic anemia. The authors suggest that the effect of the drug is on the transport of the vitamin across the ileal mucosa, though there was no evidence of ileal mucosal damage. An alternative explanation is that the vitamin B_{12} malabsorption is due to pancreatic injury and disease both by the metformin and by diabetes, for which the drug is administered (35).

Therapeutic drugs that cause mucosal damage leading to reversible malabsorption include neomycin, colchicine, para-aminosalicylic acid, methyldopa, and methotrexate (36). Methotrexate causes acute malabsorption due to cytotoxicity secondary to impaired DNA synthesis. Chronic administration of methotrexate can cause megaloblastic changes in the gut, due to folacin deficiency, and this condition can cause malabsorption of other nutrients (37), including fat and calcium.

Drug-Induced Nonenterogeneous Malabsorption Due to Bile Acid Sequestrants

Drugs that sequester bile salts, including cholestyramine and colestipol, can induce malabsorption of fats and fat-soluble vitamins which require bile salts for their optimal absorption. However, in the clinical management of hypercholesterolemic patients with these drugs, overt signs of vitamin A, D, E, and K deficiency have very seldom been reported.

Chronic pancreatitis is associated with exocrine insufficiency with a variable degree of maldigestion and malabsorption. In France, where chronic pancreatitis is more common that in the United States, alcohol abuse is the prime etiological factor. As a result of drug-induced pancreatitis, alcoholics who consume a high-fat, high-protein diet are at special risk (38). Gross steatorrhea is a late manifestation of the disease, but it does not occur until 95% of the exocrine function of the pancreas is lost (39).

Pancreatitis has been reported as a complication of azathioprine, thiazide, estrogen, furosemide, corticosteroid, tetracycline, and phenoformin therapy. However, in a 1980 critical review of case reports of pancreatitis induced by drugs (40), the authors do not allude to resultant pancreatic insufficiency leading to malabsorption. Explanations are that pancreatitis with therapeutic drugs is usually acute, leading to drug withdrawal, that with nonfatal cases the toxic pancreatitis does not cause massive loss of exocrine function, and that acute care of patients has had a greater priority than assessment of absorptive function.

In laboratory rodents, including both mice and rats, preliminary studies have shown that multiple drug insults to the pancreas, for example, with alloxan and a biguanide such as phenformin, can cause loss of exocrine and endocrine function and that chemical evidence of nutrient malabsorption can result.

SUMMARY AND CONCLUSION

From our present state of knowledge of drug effects on nutrient absorption, we are able to conclude that drugs may promote, retard, or inhibit nutrient uptake. Drug-nutrient interactions can be intraluminal and direct, or extraluminal with indirect influence of the drug on nutrient absorption. We have learned that drug-induced malabsorption becomes symptomatic and causes nutritional deficiencies with chronic use of drugs that have the potential to cause malabsorption, or with abuse of such drugs.

Finally, we are impressed by predisposing factors, which include the disease for which the drug is administered, the time at which the drug is taken, alcohol intake, and preexistent malnutrition, and which can contribute to the etiology of the malabsorption state.

REFERENCES

1. R. R. Levine, *Pharmacology. Drug Actions and Reactions,* 2nd edition, Little, Brown, Boston, 1978, p. 17.
2. M. Gibaldi, *Biopharmaceutics and Clinical Pharmacokinetics,* Lea and Febiger, Philadelphia, 1977.
3. F. H. Wilson, *Intestinal Absorption,* Saunders, Philadelphia, London, 1962.
4. G. Wiseman, *Absorption from the Intestine,* Academic, London and New York, 1964.

5. F. P. Brooks, *Control of Gastrointestinal Function*, Macmillan Co.-Collier-Macmillan Ltd., London, 1970, pp. 99–147.

6. M. Winick, Ed., *Nutrition and Gastroenterology*, Wiley, New York, 1980.

7. R. C. Rose, *Ann. Rev. Physiol.*, **42**, 157 (1980).

8. C. H. Halsted, A. Reisenauer, C. Back, and G. S. Gotterer, *J. Nutr.*, **106**, 485 (1976).

9. J. A. Blair, A. J. Matty, and A. Razzaque, *J. Physiol. Lond.*, **250**, 221 (1975).

10. G. J. Dhar, J. Selhub, C. Gay, and I. Rosenberg, *Gastroenterology*, **72**, 1049 (Abstr.) (1977).

11. S. K. Chapman, B. C. Greene, and R. R. Strieff, *J. Chromatogr.*, **145**, 302 (1978).

12. W. J. Jusko, and G. Levy, *J. Pharmacol. Sci.*, **56**, 58 (1967).

13. J. B. Houston and G. Levy, *J. Pharm. Sci.*, **64**, 1504 (1975).

14. D. A. Roe, K. Wrick, D. McLain et al., *Fed. Proc.*, **37**, 756 (Abstr.) (1978).

15. B. Stripp, *Acta Pharmacol. Toxicol.*, **22**, 353 (1965).

16. A. C. Curtis and R. S. Baliner, *J. Am. Med. Assoc.*, **113**, 1785 (1939).

17. R. J. West, and J. K. Lloyd, *Gut*, **16**, 95 (1975).

18. M. Lotz, E. Zisman, and F. C. Bartter, *New Engl. J. Med.*, **278**, 409 (1968).

19. W. L. Bloom and D. Flinchum, *J. Am. Med. Assoc.*, **174**, 1327 (1960).

20. A. Benn, C. H. J. Swan, W. T. Cooke, J. A. Blair, A. J. Matty, and M. E. Smith, *Br. Med. J.*, **1**, 148 (1971).

21. R. Carmel, et al., *Gastroenterology*, **56**, 548 (1969).

22. I. P. Palva, S. J. Salokannel, T. Timonen and H. L. A. Palva, *Acta Med. Scand.* **191**, 355 (1972).

23. J. E. McGuigan, *Gastroenterology*, **80**, 181 (1980).

24. J. H. Cummings, et al., *Br. Med. J.*, **1**, 537 (1974).

25. B. Frame, H. L. Guiang, H. M. Frost, and W. A. Reynolds, *Arch. Intern. Med.*, **128**, 794 (1971).

26. T. F. Race, I. C. Paes, and W. W. Faloon, *Am. J. Med. Sci.*, **259**, 32 (1970).

27. Y. Israel, I. Salazar, and E. Rosenmann, *J. Nutr.*, **96**, 499 (1968).

28. N. Krasner, K. M. Cochran, R. I. Russell, H. A. Carmichael, and G. G. Thompsen, *Gut*, **17**, 245 (1976).

29. J-R. Malagelada, P. Owe, and W. G. Linsheer, *Dig. Dis.*, **19**, 1016 (1974).

30. P. A. Tomasulo, R. M. H. Keter, and F. L. Iber, *Am. J. Clin. Nutr.*, **21**, 1340 (1968).

31. C. H. Halsted, E. A. Robles, and E. Mezey, *Gastroenterology*, **64**, 526 (1973).

32. J. A. Hermos, W. H. Adams, Y. K. Liu, L. W. Sullivan, and J. S. Trier, *Ann. Intern. Med.*, **76**, 957 (1972).

33. W. Perlow, E. Baraona, and C. S. Lieber, *Gastroenterology*, **72**, 680 (1977).

34. J. L. Franklin and I. H. Rosenberg, *Gastroenterology*, **64**, 517 (1973).

35. T. S. Callaghan, D. R. Hadden, and G. H. Tomkin, *Br. Med. J.*, **280**, 1214 (1980).

36. D. A. Roe, *Med. Clin. N. Amer.*, **63**, 985 (1979).

37. A. W. Craft, A. G. M. Kay, and V. N. Lawson, et al., *Br. Med. J.*, **2**, 1511 (1977).

38. H. Sarles, *Ann. N.Y. Acad. Sci.*, **252**, 171 (1975).

39. I. A. P. Bouchier, *Gastroenterology*, 2nd edition, Baillier Tindall, London, 1977, pp. 312–316.

40. A. Mallory and F. Kern, *Gastroenterology*, **78**, 813 (1980).

10

Appetite Regulation by Drugs and Endogenous Substances

A. C. SULLIVAN, Ph.D., J. TRISCARI, Ph.D., and L. CHENG

Hoffman-La Roche Inc., Nutley, New Jersey

The balance between energy intake and energy expenditure is a finely regulated system in most animals. When these regulatory controls are perturbed so as to increase intake or decrease expenditure the result is often an increase in body weight. Obesity affects a large and increasing percentage of the populations of most industrialized nations. There appear to be a number of causal and contributory factors, including genetic, metabolic, psychosocial, and environmental influences, which individually or in combination act on the energy equilibrium that must be maintained in order to prevent weight from increasing. Whatever the cause of the obesity, it is clear that obese patients are at greater risk for cardiovascular disease, stroke, and diabetes, as well as increased mortality. Because the medical and social consequences of obesity place such a heavy burden on this patient population, a great deal of thought and study has been directed toward modifying the energy equation in obese patients through reduction in caloric intake. Classically this has been accomplished by low-calorie diets or starvation regimens, and more recently through surgical procedures such as jejunoileal (or other gastrointestinal) bypass operations and gastroplasty. However, since some obese individuals gain weight even when they consume a normal caloric intake, considerable interest is being focused currently on the metabolic control of obesity, i.e., mechanisms to reduce weight by increasing caloric output or decreasing energy storage. Some aspects of this topic have been addressed in recent reviews (1–3).

The use of drugs for the control of appetitie in obese patients has been hampered by a lack of knowledge about mechanisms responsible for the regulation of food intake and also by the use of amphetamine-like compounds which are both habit forming and likely to result in the development of tolerance. Perhaps as the result of the close association between drug therapy and amphetamines, long-term drug treatment has not been seriously considered as a therapeutic approach, although such treatment is necessary to provide lasting efficacy. Until drugs are developed which have little or no addictive potential and suppress food intake without the development of tolerance, long-term treatment will not be possible.

This chapter will focus on the regulation of food intake by agents that act directly on the central nervous system or peripherally on metabolic pathways which regulate energy flow and thus may indirectly affect food intake. Several neuroregulators have been implicated in the control of food intake and recently a number of neuropeptides have also been shown to affect feeding behavior. Adrenergic, dopaminergic, serotonergic, gabanergic, peptidergic, purinergic, and opiate control mechanisms will be discussed as will a number of peripheral mechanisms that affect food intake by modifying gastric emptying, peripheral cholinergic pathways, lipid and carbohydrate metabolism, and intestinal absorption.

APPETITE SUPPRESSANTS WITH A CENTRAL ACTION

The use of anorectic agents as an adjunct to dietary restriction of caloric intake remains the only mode of pharmacotherapy available to clinicians. All of the currently available anorectic agents in the United States, with the exception of mazindol, are phenethylamine derivatives. Among these, amphetamine and its analogs (metamphetamine, phenmetrazine, phenylpropanolamine, phendimetrazine, benzphetamine, chlorphentermine, clortermine, diethylpropion, and phentermine) are structurally similar to catecholamines. Fenfluramine has a trifluoromethyl group on the phenyl ring. Several reviews have dealt with the clinical use of these agents (4–7). All of these drugs are controlled substances with different degrees of abuse potential and are subject to the regulations of the Drug Enforcement Administration. Their side effects have been well documented, and the development of tolerance to some of the agents by both animals and man has been reported. The long-term efficacy of these substances has yet to be proven. The FDA Working Party has concluded that the available anorectic drugs are equivalent in efficacy for the treatment of refractory obesity (7). A resumption of weight gain has usually followed discontinuation of drug treatment. Although fenfluramine given to obese subjects for six months produced initial rapid weight loss, weight gain was rapid after treatment was discontinued (8). Similarly, a large dose of amphetamine produced prolonged hyperphagia and obesity in rats after a transient period of anorexia and weight loss (9).

Brain monoamines are involved in the modulation of feeding behavior (10). Interaction with central monoamine neurotransmitters has been implicated in the suppression of food intake by current anorectic agents (11–14). Experimental compounds that produce hypophagia through peripheral mechanisms have also been identified. In this chapter we shall summarize some of the pertinent findings concerning the mechanisms of action of these agents.

Suppression of Appetite Through Modulation of Central Monoamine Neurotransmitters

Catecholaminergic System. Studies in rodents using the catecholamine synthesis inhibitor α-methyl-p-tryosine showed that this compound antagonized the anorectic effects of amphetamine (15–20), but had no effect on the anorectic effect of fenfluramine (21). This indicated the involvement of catecholamines in the anorexia induced by these drugs, but did not clarify which of the catecholamines was actually implicated. Further investigations using selective catecholamine antagonists have been aimed at elucidating the differential effects of catecholamines in influencing the action of anorectic agents.

Adrenergic System. An intact noradrenergic system in the brain is required for amphetamine to exert its anorectic activity. Anatomical interventions in this system have been shown to attenuate the amphetamine-induced anorexia. In rats, selective depletion of brain norepinephrine by lesions in the brain stem noradrenergic area (22) or in the ventral noradrenergic bundle (23–25) prevented amphetamine from decreasing food intake. Similar results have been found with diethylpropion, a derivative of amphetamine (25), which has been shown to decrease energy intake in obese humans (26).

On the other hand, pharmacological intervention in the noradrenergic system did not seem to interfere with the anorectic effect of amphetamine. The use of dopamine β-hydroxylase inhibitors to selectively inhibit the synthesis of norepinephrine was found to have no effect on amphetamine-induced anorexia in rats by some workers, but not by others. Thus, FLA-63 (27) and U-14,624 (28) produced no change in the appetite suppressant effect of amphetamine, whereas disulfiram (17) attenuated the hypophagic effect. Administration of amphetamine intraperitoneally (29) or directly into the anterolateral hypothalamus (30) of rats resulted in anorexia, and this effect was abolished by treatment with the β-adrenergic blocker propranolol. Other workers (31–33), using propranolol or various other β-adrenergic blockers (e.g., pindolol, dichloroisoproterenol) as well as α-adrenergic blockers (e.g., dibenamine, phentolamine, phenoxybenzamine), found that these compounds failed to influence amphetamine anorexia in rats. These results argued against a critical role for norepinephrine in the mechanism of appetite suppression induced by amphetamine.

Recent evidence, however, provides a rationale for the involvement of the central β-adrenergic system in the appetite-suppressant effect of salbutamol, a β-adrenergic stimulant (34). After receiving increasing intraperitoneal doses of salbutamol, rats demonstrated a dose-dependent reduction in food intake. The effect was abolished by pretreatment with the β-adrenergic blockers propranolol and alprenolol administered intraperitoneally or by propranolol administered intracerebroventricularly. α-Adrenergic or serotonergic blockers failed to antagonize the anorectic effect of salbutamol. Similarly, bilateral lesions of the ventral noradrenergic bundle did not influence the appetite-suppressant effect of salbutamol. The use of salbutamol for the treatment of obesity remains to be explored.

Dopaminergic System. The use of dopamine antagonists (e.g., haloperidol, pimozide, spiroperidol, and penfluridol) or the selective depletion of brain dopamine by combined treatment with intraventricularly or intracisternally injected 6-hydroxydopamine plus a monoamine oxidase inhibitor and/or desmethylimipramine, have been found to reduce the anorectic effects of amphetamine (21,25,28,32,33,35–38), mephentermine (28), phenmetrazine (32), phentermine (35,38), diethylpropion (32,35,38), DITA (20), and mazindol (19,32,33,35,38) in rodents. These studies support the importance of dopamine in mediating the anorectic effects of these drugs. On the other hand, Sanghvi et al. (29) found that haloperidol failed to prevent the anorectic effect of amphetamine. In man, a small dose of pimozide had no significant effect on dextroamphetamine-induced anorexia (39). Thus, inconsistencies exist with respect to a dopaminergic mechanism in the inhibition of eating induced by amphetamine. A lack of agreement about the involvement of dopamine in the appetite suppressant action of diethylpropion was found in the study by Borsini

et al. (25), who showed that penfluridol did not reduce the drug's anorectic effect in rats.

Recent studies have shown that the ergot derivatives lisuride,
lergotrile, and bromocriptine, as well as a dopamine receptor agonist,
piribedil, and an inhibitor of the catecholamine reuptake mechanism,
nomifensine, are potential anorectic agents with a central dopaminergic
mechanism of action; all were antagonized by pimozide. The ergot derivatives were more potent than amphetamine and fenfluramine with
respect to anorectic activity, and had less stimulatory activity than amphetamine (40,41).

Levo-DOPA produced considerable weight loss in Parkinsonian patients after prolonged treatment (42). This compound also reduced food
intake in rats (29,36,43). This effect was attenuated by treatment with
the dopamine antagonists haloperidol and spiroperidol, as well as with
the β-adrenergic antagonist propranolol, indicating that both the
adrenergic and dopaminergic systems were involved in the reduction of
food intake by levo-DOPA. However, recent studies have shown that
levo-DOPA was able to maintain weight loss in rats without causing anorexia (44,45).

Serotonergic System.   The integrity of the central serotonergic system
is of critical importance for fenfluramine to exert its anorectic effect.
This distinguishes the mechanism of action of fenfluramine from that of
all the other anorectic agents mentioned above. Fenfluramine is also
unique in that it is devoid of a central stimulant effect. Evidence
accumulating for more than a decade has strongly supported the hypothesis of a serotonergic involvement in fenfluramine-induced anorexia. This was based mainly on studies that showed an attenuation of
the inhibitory effect of fenfluramine on eating in rats after pharmacological or anatomical intervention of the serotonergic system. Serotonin
antagonists such as methergoline (21,32,46–48), methysergide (21,49),
cinanserin (21), and cyproheptadine (21) antagonized the anorexigenic
action of fenfluramine, as did the neuronal serotonin uptake inhibitor
chlorimipramine (21,47,48,50,51), and the serotonin synthesis inhibitor
p-chlorophenylalanine (28). Depletion of serotonin in the brain by
means of 5,6-dihydroxytryptamine (52) or p-chloroamphetamine (51),
as well as electrolytic lesion of the midbrain raphe, an area rich in
serotonin neurons (35), also antagonized the appetite-suppressant action
of fenfluramine. Conflicting findings have been reported for
methysergide (47), 5,-6-dihydroxytryptamine and raphe lesions (53),
p-chlorophenylalanine (46,51,53), and p-chloroamphetamine (54).

These conflicting results, however, did not offer a strong argument to refute the more compelling evidence supporting the importance of the serotonergic system in the mechanism of action of fenfluramine. It has also been shown that d-fenfluramine, a serotonin releaser and uptake inhibitor, caused a significant reduction of [^{3}H]serotonin binding sites in rat cortex (55).

Fenfluramine analogs with anorectic activity have been identified (33) (for review see Refs. 56,77). Some of them have demonstrated clinical efficacy.

Other compounds known to inhibit serotonin uptake or to act as serotonin agonists have been shown to reduce food intake in rats. Included in this group are quipazine (57,58), MK-212 (6-chloro-2-(1-piperzinyl)-pyrazine) (59,60), and meta-chlorophenylpiperazine (55,61). Pretreatment with methergoline attenuated the hypophagic effects of these agents, suggesting a similar mechanism of action to that of fenfluramine.

Zimelidine is an antidepressant with an inhibitory effect on serotonin uptake. A recent double-bind, placebo-controlled study with zimelidine in obese subjects showed that this drug produced a small but significant decrease in body weight and appetite (62). The anorectic action of RU 25591   (6,7,8,9-tetrahydro   N,N-dimethyl   5-[4-nitrophenyl]oxy 5H-benzocyclohepten 7-amine, cis-fumarate) demonstrated in rats, dogs, and pigs could be partially explained by its selective ability to block serotonin uptake (63).

Role of GABA.   Evidence has been accumulating implicating a role for gamma-aminobutyric acid (GABA) in the neural control of hunger and satiety (64,65). Enhancement or suppression of ingestive behavior has been demonstrated through differentially modulating GABA levels in specific brain sites by local injections of GABA (66), the antagonists bicuculline methiode and picrotoxin (67,68), or the GABA agonist muscimol (69,70). The irreversible GABA-transaminase inhibitor ethanolamine-O-sulfate produced a sustained decrease in food intake and body weight in rats after intracisternal injection (71). The decrease in food intake was accompanied by elevations of GABA levels in the brain and reduction of brain GABA transaminase activity. Whereas administration of muscimol intracerebroventricularly (70) or into the ventromedial hypothalamus (69) induced feeding in rats, intraperitoneal injection of the same compound produced a decrease in milk consumption (71).

The studies discussed above offer a rationale for developing orally active anorectic agents acting on the GABA-ergic system. Oral administration of GABA in the diet decreased body weight and food intake in rats (72) and mice (73). Genetically obese (ob/ob) mice were less sensitive than lean mice to GABA. The GABA analog THIP (4,5,6,7-tetrahydro-isoxazolo[5,4-c]pyridin-3-ol) produced a dose-dependent decrease in food consumption after oral administration in rats (74). This anorectic action was blocked by pretreatment with bicuculline, supporting the involvement of GABA receptors. The oral administration of BW 357U (1-(n-decyl)-3-pyrazolidinone), a potent, irreversible inhibitor of GABA transaminase, resulted in a decrease in body weight and food consumption in rats (75). Decreases in body weight were directly correlated with increases in brain GABA levels. Decreased appetite was specifically correlated with a twofold increase in GABA levels in the hypothalamus (76). However, toxicity precluded testing this compound in man. Modulation of brain GABA levels offers an attractive approach to the development of novel anorectic agents.

Peripheral Effects of Central Anorectic Agents

In addition to suppression of food consumption, effects on peripheral energy metabolism have also been demonstrated for some of the anorectic agents (for review see Refs. 56,77,78). However, it is not clear at present whether these metabolic effects are contributory to the antiobesity activity of these agents, since the metabolic effects occurred at concentrations ten to 100 times greater than therapeutic doses (79).

Fenfluramine and several of its derivatives decreased the synthesis of triglycerides by rat liver (80) and human adipose tissue (81) in vitro and rabbit liver in vivo (82). These effects were attributed to the inhibition of phosphatidate phosphohydrolase (80). An inhibition of the intestinal absorption of triglycerides has been demonstrated in rats (83–85), and this effect was believed to be due to the inhibition of intestinal palmitoyl-CoA:monoolein acyltransferase (85,86) or pancreatic lipase (84,87,88). Fenfluramine and amphetamine reduced lipogenesis and cholesterogenesis by rats both in vitro and in vivo (84). It has also been reported that fenfluramine had no influence on the rates of lipogenesis in liver and adipose tissue in obese mice (89). Marked decreases of serum triglycerides and cholesterol have also been observed with fenfluramine in diabetic and hyperlipidemic patients (90).

Mazindol administered to obese subjects produced a significant reduction in serum triglycerides and cholesterol, and a significant elevation of nonesterified fatty acids (91,92). Hydroxyacyl CoA dehydrogenase activity in striated muscle was elevated, whereas malic dehydrogenase was decreased (92).

Fenfluramine, norfenfluramine, or flutiorex significantly increased glucose uptake by isolated rat hemidiaphragm (93) (Kirby and Turner, 1975) and human skeletal muscle (94,95). Similar results have been shown for mazindol and ciclazindol (96–98). Fenfluramine (99) and mazindol (100), respectively, inhibited the specific binding of insulin to human adipose tissue and rat isolated fat cells; glucose oxidation was enhanced by fenfluramine and abolished by mazindol. Insulin sensitivity in vivo was improved in obese mice given doses of fenfluramine which did not induce weight loss, demonstrating an effect of this drug distinct from its anorexigenic properties (89). Fenfluramine (101) and mazindol (102) improved glucose tolerance in diabetics and obese subjects, respectively.

Involvement of Purines

Recently, purines have been implicated in the endogenous regulation of food intake (103). The purine inosine, administered intraperitoneally, was found to suppress several models of food intake in rats. These models included feeding induced by the benzodiazepine diazepam, and the GABA agonist muscimol. That benzodiazepines have an appetite-enhancing effect has been confirmed by various workers. The role of GABA in modulating ingestive behavior has been discussed previously. In addition, it has been suggested that GABA may be involved in the mechanism of action of benzodiazepine-induced feeding. Inosine and hypoxanthine have been identified as possible endogenous ligands that compete with benzodiazepines for binding to receptor sites. Interestingly, 2-deoxyguanosine and 2-deoxyinosine also suppressed food deprivation-induced feeding, as did inosine. On the other hand, 7-methylinosine, a purine that does not bind to the benzodiazepine receptor in vitro, did not have an anorectic effect under the same experimental conditions. These data suggest that purines may act as satiety factors by having a role in the central regulation of appetite through interaction with the benzodiazepine receptor.

Suppression of Appetite Through Modulation of Endorphins

Cumulative evidence suggests that endogenous opiate peptides are involved in the regulation of ingestive behavior. Elevated levels of β-endorphin have been found in the pituitaries of genetically obese mice and rats and might be involved in the development of hyperphagia and obesity in these animals (104,105). β-Endorphin, whether injected intracerebroventricularly (106) or into the ventromedial hypothalamus (69) of rats, stimulated food intake. A recently isolated opiate peptide, dynorphin-(1–13), had the same effect, which could be antagonized by naloxone (107). A large number of studies have demonstrated that the opiate antagonist naloxone reduced food intake in normal and obese rats, for example (104,108,109). Recently, it was found that a long-acting derivative, zinc tannate of naloxone, reduced hyperphagia and increased energy expenditure in rats with diet-induced obesity (110). Overeating induced by various types of stress (i.e., tail-pinch, 2-deoxy-D-glucose, food deprivation) and nighttime food intake were inhibited by the administration of naloxone (70,111,112). A similar attenuating effect was found after the administration of dexamethasone, a glucocorticoid which inhibits the synthesis and stress-induced release of pituitary β-endorphin (113). The above results suggest that opiate antagonists may have therapeutic importance as anorectics selective for stress-induced hyperphagia. However, other studies have found that naloxone did not suppress tail-pinch-induced eating (114), and that naltrexone had no effect on food intake or deprivation-induced feeding (115) in rats.

The effect of naloxone has been evaluated in patients with the Prader-Willi syndrome (116). These patients characteristically overeat and are massively obese. Of three patients treated with naloxone, food intake was reduced in the two males with abnormally high baseline consumption. No effect was observed in the female patient, whose food consumption was less excessive. Although only a small pilot study, the results lend support to the suggestion based on animal studies that opiate antagonists may have therapeutic application in the treatment of hyperphagia and obesity.

Suppression of Appetite Through Modulation of the Neuroendocrine System

Thyrotropin releasing hormone (TRH) is a central neuropeptide that decreased food intake in food deprived rats (117,118) and lean and obese Zucker rats (105) whether injected intraperitoneally or intraventricularly. A smaller dosage was required to elicit hypophagia when TRH was injected into the brain, suggesting a central site of action (118). TRH also suppressed stress-induced hyperphagia in rats upon intraventricular or subcutaneous administration (119). Intraventricular administration of D-Ala-Met-Enkephalin reversed the anorectic effect of TRH, suggesting an involvement of brain enkephalins in the mechanism of action of TRH. The anorectic effect of TRH was attributed to the metabolic breakdown product histidyl-proline-diketropiperazine (cyclo-(His-Pro)), since the latter was also able to suppress stress-induced eating, starvation-induced eating, and spontaneous eating in rats (120). The action of cyclo-(His-Pro) was more potent than that of TRH, and was also antagonized by D-Ala-met-Enkephalin. It was postulated that TRH acted as pro-hormone for cyclo-(His-Pro), and that cyclo-(His-Pro) may be a central neuromodulator of appetite control.

Calcitonin suppressed appetite in rats after subcutaneous or intracerebral injections (121). Smaller doses were required when calcitonin was injected intracerebroventricularly. Calcitonin also suppressed stress-induced eating and calcium chloride-induced eating in rats (122). In monkeys, calcitonin produced a 90% reduction in feeding (123). The suppression of food intake was maintained over three to five days. When calcitonin was given to psychiatric patients, it produced a modest loss in body weight. It was speculated that endogenous calcitonin was involved in the regulation of feeding behavior by acting directly on the central nervous system, possibly through an alteration in calcium metabolism in neuronal tissue.

Satietin is a highly potent anorexigenic glycopeptide isolated from human serum as well as sera of several other species (124,125). It produced a dose-dependent decrease in food consumption in starved rats whether administered intravenously, subcutaneously, orally, or intracerebroventricularly. Satietin was devoid of any of the behavioral or physiological effects exhibited by amphetamine or fenfluramine. Thus it appeared that satietin had a unique action in that it selectively inhibited food intake. These results led to the hypothesis that satietin acted directly on the central regulation of feeding through its role as a satiety signal.

Substance P suppressed stress-induced eating (using the mild tail-pinch model), but not starvation-induced eating in rats after parenteral administration (126). This effect was possibly associated with the role of substance P in the modulation of pain transmission. Intraventricular administration of somatostatin has produced anorexia (117). Intracerebroventricular injection of spermine, a polyamine that is widely distributed in the brain, suppressed feeding and drinking behavior in satiated rats (127). These findings suggest that spermine may play some functional role in the brain involving the modulation of hunger and satiety.

APPETITE SUPPRESSANTS WITH A PERIPHERAL SITE OF ACTION

Agents Acting on the Gastrointestinal System

Gastrointestinal Hormones as Satiety Factors.   Several gastrointestinal peptide hormones have been reported to inhibit feeding. Among these, cholecystokinin (CCK) is the most extensively studied (for review see (128)). Interest in bombesin is also increasing (119,129,130). The fact that both CCK and bombesin could also inhibit sham feeding in rats without causing toxic effects indicates that they may function as short-term satiety signals to regulate the cessation of eating.

There is now substantial evidence that CCK inhibits feeding in several animal species. Recently, the C-terminal octapeptide of CCK (CCK-8) has been found to decrease food intake in lean (131,132) and obese (133) adults, confirming results obtained in obese mice (134) and obese rats (135). These results indicate that CCK-8 may have potential use as an appetite suppressant in the treatment of obesity. Trypsin inhibitors such as trasylol and N,N-diemthyl-carbamoylmethyl 4-(4-guanidinoben-zoyloxy)-phenyl acetate methanesulfate (DCGPM) decreased meal size in Zucker obese rats. Chronic administration of DCGPM also reduced daily food intake and body weight in obese rats. Trypsin inhibitors are postulated to exert these effects through increasing CCK release (136).

There are now conflicting reports concerning a role for brain CCK in the etiology of obesity. CCK-8 is present in rat brain (137). It has been suggested that low brain levels of CCK-8 may be responsible for the hyperphagia of genetically obese (ob/ob) mice, since these mice had significantly lower CCK-8 content in the cerebral cortex compared to their nonobese littermates and normal mice (138). Consistent with these findings is the observation that CCK receptors were significantly increased in the cerebral cortex of obese Zucker rats and obese (ob/ob) mice compared to their lean littermates (139). The reduced CCK concentration in obese rodents was thought to be due to an increase in the binding of CCK to brain receptors. Furthermore, obese mice and rats were less sensitive than their lean counterparts to the satiety effects of CCK-8 (134,135). On the other hand, several studies failed to show that obesity in rodents was associated with reduced CCK concentrations in the brain (140–142).

Considerable controversy also exists as to whether CCK induces satiety via a central or a peripheral mechanism. In addition to being present in rodent brains as mentioned above, CCK was also found in the cerebrospinal fluid of humans (143). Continuous injections of CCK-8 at 0.01 pmoles/min into the cerebral ventricles of sheep produced hypophagia (144), whereas continuous intravenous injections of 2.55 pmoles/min did not affect food ingestion (145). Injections of CCK antibody (146) or the CCK antagonist dibutyryl cyclic GMP (147) into the cerebral ventricles of sheep stimulated feeding. In addition, injections of CCK intraperitoneally or into the hypothalamus of rats abolished the feeding response to centrally administered norepinephrine; a higher dose was required when CCK was administered intraperitoneally (148). These studies support the hypothesis that CCK acts centrally to elicit satiety. On the other hand, in the model of tail pinch-induced eating in rats, the minimal effective dose of CCK in suppressing appetitive behavior was smaller after peripheral than after central administration, suggesting a peripheral mechanism of action for CCK (149). Although CCK appears to produce satiety via both central and peripheral mechanisms, the prevailing evidence favors a peripheral action for CCK (128,150).

Anorectic Agents That Inhibit Gastric Emptying.   It has been postulated that the control of appetite is mediated partly through the control of gastric emptying and that increased food consumption may be positively correlated with rapid transfer of energy in the gastric content from the stomach to the duodenum (151). Slowing of gastric emptying has been suggested as a means of producing therapeutic anorexia (152).

(−)-*threo*-Chlorocitric acid is a novel anorectic agent that suppressed food intake in dogs and in lean and obese rats when administered at low doses (153). This compound also significantly inhibited gastric emptying, and this effect was suggested to be, at least in part, responsible for its anorectic effect (154). A similar effect was reported for the structurally related (± -)-*threo*-epoxyaconitic acid (155). A positive relationship was shown between the potent anorectic effect of this agent and its ability to slow the rate of energy transfer from the stomach to the duodenum.

The naloxone-induced reduction in food intake in patients with Prader-Willi syndrome (116) has been discussed previously. Since naloxone given intravenously to human volunteers significantly delayed gastric emptying of a test meal, it was suggested that this opiate antagonist suppressed caloric intake by causing gastric retention rather than by its effect on hypothalamic or pituitary β-endorphin activity (156). On the other hand, naloxone given as a continuous intravenous infusion to human subjects failed to inhibit gastric emptying of polyethylene glycol incorporated into an amino acid meal (157). In contrast, morphine significantly delayed gastric emptying. The enkephalin analog d-Ala^2, MePhe^4, Met (O)-ol-enkephalin (DAMME, Sandoz FK 33-824) significantly inhibited gastric emptying in healthy volunteers (158). DAMME caused a sensation of heaviness in the legs, abdomen, and thorax. However, its effect on food consumption was not reported.

Several agents that have been reported to reduce food intake were also found to inhibit gastric emptying. These include salbutamol (159), levo-DOPA (160), and spermine (161). A relationship between satiety and inhibition of gastric emptying was also demonstrated in a study of the three sugars glucose, D-xylose, and fructose (162). The anorectic effects of CCK-8 have been discussed in the previous section. Whereas CCK-8 was found to cause dose-related inhibition of gastric emptying in the dog by acting on both the pylorus and the proximal stomach (163), studies with suckling rats showed that CCK-8 significantly depressed food intake without slowing gastric emptying, indicating a lack of correlation between the rate of gastric emptying and the regulation of satiety (164). Caerulein is structurally related to CCK and has been found to delay gastric emptying of solids in man (165). Another gastrointestinal hormone, bombesin, has been reported to delay gastric emptying in rats (166).

Other Agents.   A new appetite-reducing preparation of hydrophilic granules (Prefil), given as an adjunct to dietary restriction, resulted in a significantly greater weight loss in obese subjects when compared with diet control alone (167). Prefil consists of flavored granules containing almost 60% dietary fiber as vegetable gums. When taken with water before a meal, the granules swell in the stomach to cause a sensation of fullness and satiety conducive to reduction of food intake.

Gallic acid administered to rats through systemic infusions or intragastric intubations significantly reduced their food intake (168). Propyl gallate was more potent than gallic acid. Propyl gallate may modify the taste of food. Although the effect of gallic acid on food intake was not entirely mediated through taste aversion, the role of taste in the overall effect of gallic acid could not be excluded.

Cholinergic Involvement in Appetite Regulation

The involvement of a peripheral cholinergic mechanism in feeding behavior was suggested by studies in which the intraperitoneal administration of the centrally inactive cholinergic antagonists atropine methyl nitrate and scopolamine methyl nitrate suppressed food intake without affecting water intake. In those studies the centrally active cholinergic antagonists atropine and scopolamine also suppressed food intake following intraperitoneal administration but, in addition, they decreased water intake (169). These studies suggested that while central cholinergic pathways are definitely involved in water intake, food intake regulation may depend to some extent on peripheral cholinergic mechanisms. The effect of peripherally acting anticholinergic agents was shown to be separate not only from the central cholinergic effect on water intake, but also from several other behavioral responses such as biting, swallowing, or licking. The intraperitoneal administration of atropine methyl nitrate produced a dose-dependent suppression of sham feeding of a liquid diet, but had no effect on sham drinking of water on the above-mentioned behavioral responses (170). Chronic administration of atropine sulfate to 23-hour food deprived rats suppressed food intake throughout the treatment period, suggesting a lack of development of tolerance to the drug (171).

Additional evidence that peripheral cholinergic mechanisms might be involved in the regulation of food intake comes from studies in which subdiaphragmatic vagotomies were performed in previously ventromedial hypothalamic (VMH) lesioned rats. This surgical denervation of the viscera resulted in a reversal of the hyperphagia and obesity commonly associated with VMH lesions (172). It was postulated that: (a) perhaps the elimination of efferent signals to peripheral organs such as the pancreas prevented the induction of hyperinsulinemia in VMH lesioned rats and thus reduced the hyperphagia, or that (b) the termination of afferent feedback from such organs as the liver or stomach resulted in a disruption of the feeding pattern. However, recent studies suggest that the vagal involvement in feeding behavior may not be completely mediated through cholinergic mechanisms or at least not those systems sensitive to scopolamine methyl nitrate (173). The administration of scopolamine methyl nitrate to VMH lesioned rats significantly decreased food intake during the first three weeks of treatment, but was ineffective during the last three weeks of treatment. Moreover, if treatment with the anticholinergic agent was initiated three weeks prior to the production of the lesions, the hyperphagia induced by the lesions could not be prevented (173).

Another experimental approach to determining the extent of cholinergic involvement in the regulation of food intake behavior has been to elicit feeding by electrically stimulating the lateral hypothalamic area by means of implanted electrodes. The threshold for stimulation-induced feeding can be lowered by the intraperitoneal administration of physostigmine, a cholinesterase inhibitor, and reversed by the intraperitoneal administration of atropine (174), or it can be increased by subdiaphragmatic vagotomy (175). The administration of centrally acting atropine had no independent effect on the stimulation-induced feeding in either study. In the first study (174) it was argued that since the animals were satiated prior to testing, their cholinergic activity was low and therefore blocking cholinergic receptors with atropine would not be expected to produce any effect on stimulation-induced feeding. In the second study (175) the argument posed was that atropine sulfate selectively blocks efferent responses and that the disruption of eating behaviors resulting from vagotomy is the result of the elimination of afferent feedback. This latter argument suggests a peripheral cholinergic involvement in the control of feeding which is consistent with the observation that cholinergic agents may not have a potent central effect on food intake.

The direct application of crystalline acetylcholine carbachol or muscarine to the hypothalami of rats resulted in increased water intake without altering food intake (176). However, this early work does not agree with more recent studies in rabbits. Food intake was increased in a dose-dependent manner by the intrahypothalamic injection of carbachol in rabbits (177), but water intake was decreased at equipotent doses of carbachol which increased food intake. Further evidence for a possible central cholinergic involvement in feeding behavior comes from studies in which antibodies to nicotinic acetylcholine receptor were injected intracerebroventricularly each day in rabbits to produce a potent suppression of food intake (178). The discrepancies between the earlier and more recent studies may be due to species or methodological differences. Despite these two last-mentioned studies in rabbits, the weight of the evidence appears to support a peripheral cholinergic component in the control of feeding behavior. Furthermore, if there is any central cholinergic involvement, it may be specific to one or more discrete areas of the brain. This is suggested by studies in which the intraventricular administration of β-endorphin or enkephalins resulted in increased hippocampal (179) but decreased cortical levels (180) of acetylcholine. These effects were reversed by naloxone in the cortex but not in the hippocampus. Considering the role of endorphin and naloxone on food intake, the effects produced in both the cortex and the hippocampus are not entirely consistent with a central cholinergic mechanism for the effect of these compounds on food intake. The possible involvement of peripheral cholinergic pathways in feeding behavior promises another pharmacological avenue to the control of food intake. However, control of food intake through the modulation of central cholinergic pathways would need to be approached with caution in view of the association between decreased central cholinergic function and Alzheimer's disease (181).

Metabolic Agents

Hydroxycitrate. (−)-Hydroxycitrate is an inhibitor of ATP: citrate lyase (182), the enzyme that cleaves citrate to produce the extramitochondrial precursor of fatty acid synthesis, acetyl CoA. Although the inhibition of this enzymatic pathway limits the availability of carbon precursors for fatty acid synthesis (183,184), the fate of the unutilized carbons is not entirely clear. However, it has been postulated (1,2) that the increased hepatic concentrations of glucose-6-phosphate and fructose-6-phosphate and the decreased concentrations of glycolytic intermediates (185) may signal increased glycogen synthesis (186), which may in turn suppress food intake. The increased hepatic glycogen synthesis and glycogen levels following hydroxycitrate treatment could conceivably activate hepatic energy- or gluco-receptors. The central processing of this information would in turn lead to the determination that caloric intake sufficient to restore body energy stores has been accomplished and thus that food intake should be terminated.

Hydroxycitrate inhibited food intake in lean (187) and obese (188) rats, mice (189), and chickens (190). Food intake was suppressed in a dose-dependent fashion following 30 days of intragastric drug administration (187). The hydroxycitrate-induced anorexia was probably not the result of a direct central effect, since negligible amounts of labeled hydroxycitrate were found in the brains of treated rats (Triscari and Sullivan, unpublished observations). Furthermore, the suppression of food intake in rats did not require an intact hypothalamus, since hydroxycitrate suppressed food intake in rats with VMH lesions as well as sham controls (189).

When hydroxycitrate was given to mature Sprague Dawley rats as a dietary admix, food intake was suppressed during the first seven but not the last seven weeks of treatment (189). Despite this apparent normalization of food intake during the latter stages of the experimental treatment period, there was no overeating or compensation for the earlier reduction in food intake. Overeating was also not observed in lean and obese Zucker rats during a 38- to 39-day treatment period or an additional 49-day recovery period during which the rate of growth of previously treated rats increased 1.3-fold to twofold (188). Therefore, although the effect of hydroxycitrate on body weight gain has been postulated to be primarily the result of a decrease in food intake, as demonstrated by equivalent changes in the weight gain and carcass lipid content of animals pair-fed to the hydroxycitrate-treated animals (187,190), the data in Zucker rats (188) suggest that hydroxycitrate may also have a small metabolic effect on weight gain independent from its anorectic activity.

The anorexia produced by hydroxycitrate is probably the result of its effect on metabolic processes. The evidence suggests that increased glycogen synthesis and/or levels produced by hydroxycitrate treatment may be closely linked to this anorectic effect. This is supported by data which demonstrate that TOFA [5-(tetradecyloxy)-2-furoic acid], which is a potent inhibitor of lipogenesis (191,192), does not suppress food intake in Sprague Dawley or lean and obese Zucker rats (193).

Biguanides.   It has been suggested that biguanides have anorectic activity (194). This is based primarily on their potential to decrease body weight gain in obese diabetic patients (195). However, it is possible that the observed metabolic effects of biguanides may contribute directly to the weight loss. The primary effect of biguanides in humans is the normalization of hyperglycemia in non-insulin-dependent diabetics. Although the mechanism for the euglycemic and weight-reducing actions of biguanides has not yet been elucidated, one possible explanation for both of these effects is the reported inhibition by phenethylbiguanide (phenformin) and butyl biguanide (Buformin) of small intestinal glucose transport in rats and humans (196–198), although this observation has been challenged (199). Another plausible explanation for the antihyperglycemic effects of biguanides is increased peripheral insulin-mediated glucose utilization (200–202) or decreased gluconeogenesis (203).

Increased glucose utilization has been recently attributed to an increase in insulin-receptor sites following dimethylbiguanide (metformin) treatment (204). Erythrocytes obtained from patients without any diabetic complications after two days of oral treatment with dimethylbiguanide demonstrated an increase in insulin-receptor number per cell. The increase was primarily due to a change in low-affinity receptor sites but there was no change in circulating insulin levels. Although butylbiguanide did not alter insulin levels in normal patients (205), dimethylbiguanide decreased both basal and glucose-induced insulin levels in obese patients (206). The decreased insulin resistance and circulating insulin levels and increased insulin-receptor number following biguanide treatment might explain both the increased peripheral glucose utilization and the decreased food intake (since hyperinsulinemia may lead to increased food intake).

In contrast to the facilitative effect of biguanides on insulin-dependent glucose metabolism, they inhibit insulin-stimulated lipoprotein lipase activity. The induction of lipoprotein lipase activity in human adipose tissue biopsies was blocked by dimethylbiguanide (207). These data suggest that biguanides may decrease fat storage in adipose tissue and may thus decrease body weight.

Delayed gastric emptying has also been suggested as a possible mechanism for biguanide action (7). As discussed previously, delayed gastric emptying is thought to be the mechanism responsible for the anorectic activity of (−)-*threo*-chlorocitric acid (154) and (± -)-*Threo*-transepoxyaconitic acid (155).

Although biguanides have been available for years, their anorectic and antiobesity effects have not been explored thoroughly because biguanide administration may result in lactic acidosis, which could prove fatal in a significant percentage of the susceptible population (208). Moreover, deaths from cardiovascular complications have been reported to be greater for phenethylbiguanide-treated patients than for controls (209), although the methodology used in these studies has been criticized (210).

Acarbose.   Following the isolation of acarbose (Bay g 5421), a complex polysaccharide that inhibits glucosidase activity (211), it was demonstrated that acarbose suppressed the postprandial elevation of glucose and insulin in humans (212) as a result of the incomplete digestion of starch or glucose meals. A twofold greater decrease in postprandial blood glucose levels following treatment with acarbose could be accomplished if the patients were given a starch diet that contained a fiber such as guar gum (213). Although the effect of guar gum might be to alter gastric emptying, acarbose by itself had no effect on gastric emptying in patients with dumping syndrome (214). In these patients acarbose improved the symptoms of dumping syndrome following a 50 g sucrose load, probably by reducing the osmotic effect of glucose in the intestine. Plasma glucose and insulin levels were much lower than those observed in controls. Since gastric inhibitory polypeptide (GIP) was also suppressed by acarbose treatment, it was postulated that the decrease in insulin was secondary to the decrease in GIP (214). In non-insulin-dependent diabetic patients there was a reduction in postprandial blood glucose levels and urinary glucose excretion (215). Thus it appears that acarbose is a potentially useful antidiabetic agent.

Acarbose was also shown to be an antiobesity agent as well as a potential hypoglycemic drug. Acarbose decreased body weight gain in obese Zucker rats in a dose-dependent manner (212), probably as a result of its inhibition of food intake in these animals (216). Inhibition of food intake was also observed in lean diabetic and control rats fed a high-starch or starch and sucrose diet but not in rats fed a high-glucose diet (217). As was observed in diabetic humans, diabetic rats fed a high-starch or starch and sucrose diet showed decreased postprandial blood glucose levels and decreased urinary excretion of glucose (217). The decreased food intake and inhibition of glucosidase activity following acarbose treatment produced lower VLDL levels in Zucker rats (216), sucrose fed rats (218, 219), and WR-1339 hypertriglyceridemic rats (219) probably as a result of decreased VLDL secretion.

An inhibitory effect of acarbose on food intake was not observed in all studies. Food intake and caloric intake were reported to be increased in acarbose-treated rats given a corn starch diet or a chow diet plus a 40% sucrose solution (220, 221). In those studies acarbose did not alter preference for sweet solutions or lever pressing for food, nor did it affect body weight gain.

Recently an α-amylase inhibitor was reported to have many of the effects observed with acarbose. Trestatin (Ro 9-0154) lowered blood glucose and insulin levels in rats and dogs following a starch load. It reversed glucose-induced hyperglycemia and the hyperglycemia and glucosuria observed in lean diabetic rats. Trestatin also decreased body weight gain in rats fed a high-starch diet (222).

Whether acarbose and trestatin decrease body weight gain as a result of their inhibition of the digestion of polysaccharides or as a result of their suppression of food intake still remains to be determined.

ANALYSIS OF MEAL PATTERNS

In the evaluation of anorectic effects of appetite suppressants, it was customary in the earlier studies to use the quantity of food consumed as a parameter of drug efficacy. In recent years, the importance of analyzing the effect of anorectic agents on the pattern of food intake is being recognized. In addition to measuring the total amount of food ingested during a given period of time, researchers have begun to dissect ingestive behavior into its individual components and to evaluate the response of each component to anorectic drugs. The components, or microstructure, of food intake consist of meal size, meal frequency, latency to feeding, rate of eating, duration of feeding, the effects of food texture, selective suppression of protein, carbohydrate, or fat consumption, and others. Such studies have enhanced our understanding of the subtle differences among various anorectic agents.

Results from a number of experiments in rats have shown the differing effects of various anorectic agents on the microstructure of food intake (223). Amphetamine, fenfluramine, and mazindol all suppressed food intake. Amphetamine increased the latency to feeding and the rate of feeding (g/min); it decreased the duration and size of feeding bouts, but produced no change in their number. Mazindol shared the property of amphetamine in increasing the rate of eating and decreasing the duration of feeding bouts, but differed from amphetamine in that it had no effect on latency to feeding or size of bouts, but decreased the number and duration of bouts. Fenfluramine, on the other hand, differed from both amphetamine and mazindol in that it alone demonstrated a decrease in the rate of eating; there was no effect on latency of feeding and the number or duration of bouts, but the size of bouts was decreased. Additional data point out that agents which induce synthesis or release of serotonin, or inhibit its reuptake, properties also shared by fenfluramine, tend to reduce meal size and the rate of eating while failing to prolong feeding latency. The characteristic effects of amphetamine and fenfluramine on certain meal pattern parameters were antagonized by the dopamine-receptor blocking agent pimozide and serotonin-receptor blocking agent methergoline, respectively (224). Spiperone is a potent dopamine-receptor antagonist. Like fenfluramine, it also retarded the rate of eating in rats (225). Pretreatment with spiperone antagonized the effect of amphetamine and mazindol to increase eating rate, to reduce duration of eating, and to prolong latency. However, spiperone enhanced the tendency of fenfluramine to reduce the rate of eating. Those studies indicate that the effects of anorectic agents on the microstructure of eating also have a neurochemical basis.

The effects of amphetamine and fenfluramine on the fine structure of eating in rats was confirmed in humans by one group (226). On the other hand, another study showed that both amphetamine and fenfluramine led to similar responses in that both increased the latency to eat and decreased the rate of eating (227).

Anorectic agents with a peripheral site of action have also been shown to affect the pattern of meal ingestion. Several studies have attempted to analyze the changes in meal pattern produced by CCK in rodents (134, 135, 228, 229). In both Zucker obese and lean rats, CCK-8 decreased meal size and the rate of eating (g/min) and increased satiety ratio (min/g); postmeal interval and the duration of eating were not changed (134, 135).

(−)-*threo*-Chlorocitric acid is a compound that depressed food intake, possibly by delaying gastric emptying. Its effects on meal patterns have been studied in obese and lean Zucker rats. (−)-*threo*-Chlorocitric acid reduced food intake by a reduction of meal size taken in the dark with no effect on meal frequency (230).

Anorectic drugs also selectively modify the intake of protein, carbohydrates, or fats. Drugs with a serotoninergic mechanism of action, such as fenfluramine, MK 212, fluoxetine, and CGP 6085, reduced carbohydrate consumption while sparing protein intake in rats (231, 232). Studies with fenfluramine in rats were confirmed in obese patients who craved carbohydrates (233). Amphetamine has been found to produce a sustained suppression of fat consumption in rats (234).

Studies on the microstructure of food intake could have important implications in the treatment of obesity, since they will possibly enable clinicians to apply anorectic drugs selectively on the basis of the type of hyperphagia manifested by the obese patient.

CONCLUSION

The control of food intake is an increasingly complex topic that has not progressed very far from the classical two-center hypothesis for the control of appetite and satiety in the brain. If such centers do exist it is clear that there are a number of pathways, both central and peripheral, which provide inputs into these centers. Since feeding behavior is so closely linked to systems that regulate energy metabolism, it is no surprise that drugs which interfere with peripheral carbohydrate or lipid metabolism should also have the potential to produce anorexia. Appetite suppressants have been used as short-term adjuncts to the treatment of obesity partly because of the tolerance that develops to these drugs (although it has recently been suggested that this is due not to tolerance but to the establishment of a new body weight set-point (235) and partly because the effect of these drugs is only slightly greater than that produced by placebo alone (see (5) for a review). Although these anorectics have been very useful in studying the mechanisms involved in appetite regulation, the long-term efficacy of such drug treatment awaits a new generation of appetite suppressants.

It is probable that some of the mechanisms described in this chapter play an important part in appetite regulation. An understanding of the molecular basis for both the peripheral and the central control of food intake should lead to the design of anorectics that will be more specific, safer, and appropriately tailored to individual needs and long-term treatment.

REFERENCES

1. A. C. Sullivan, C. Nauss-Karol, and L. Cheng, *New Directions in the Pharmacological Treatment of Obesity: I. Appetite Suppressants and Modulators of Intestinal Absorption*, in press.

2. A. C. Sullivan, C. Nauss-Karol, and L. Cheng, *New Directions in the Pharmacological Treatment of Obesity: II. Inhibitors of Lipid Synthesis, Modulators of Adipocyte Metabolism or Hormonal Function, and Thermogenic Agents*, in press.

3. J. Himms-Hagen, "Nonshivering Thermogenesis, Brown Adipose Tissue, and Obesity," in R. F. Beers, Jr. and E. G. Bassett, Eds., *Nutritional Factors: Modulating Effects of Metabolic Processes*, Raven, New York, 1981, p. 85.

4. A. C. Sullivan and L. Cheng, "Appetite Regulation and Its Modulation by Drugs," in J. N. Hathcock and J. Coon, Eds., *Nutrition and Drug Interrelations, Nutrition Foundation Monograph Series*, Academic, New York/San Francisco/London, 1978, p. 21.

5. A. C. Sullivan and K. Comai, *Int. J. Obes.*, **2**, 167 (1978).

6. J. F. Munro, *Int. J. Obes.*, **3**, 171 (1979).

7. J. G. Douglas and J. F. Munro, *Drugs*, **21**, 362 (1981).

8. A. J. Stunkard, L. W. Craighead, and R. O'Brien, *Lancet*, **2**, 1045 (1980).

9. B. G. Hoebel, L. Hernandez, A. P. Monaco, and W. C. Miller, *Life Sci.*, **28**, 77 (1981).

10. B. G. Hoebel and S. F. Leibowitz, *Res. Publ. Assoc. Res. Nerv. Ment. Dis.*, **59**, 103 (1981).

11. B. G. Hoebel, *Annu. Rev. Pharmacol. Toxicol.*, **17**, 605 (1977).

12. S. Garattini and R. Samanin, Eds., *Central Mechanisms of Anorectic Drugs*, Raven, New York, 1978.

13. B. V. Clineschmidt and P. R. Bunting, *Prog. Neuro-psychopharmacol*, **4**, 327 (1980).

14. R. Samanin, "Central Mechanisms of Anorectic Drugs," in F. G. De las Heras and S. Vega, Eds., *Medicinal Chemistry Advances*, Pergamon, Oxford/New York, 1981, p. 271.

15. A. Weissman, B. K. Koe, S. S. Tenen, *J. Pharmacol. Exp. Therap.*, **151**, 339 (1966).

16. S. G. Holtzman and R. E. Jewett, *Psychopharmacologia* (Berlin), **22**, 151 (1971).

17. H.-H. Frey and R. Schulz, *Biochem. Pharmacol.*, **22**, 3041 (1973).

18. L. A. Baez, *Psychopharmacologia* (Berlin), **35**, 91 (1974).

19. F. Zambotti, M. O. Carruba, F. Barzaghi, L. Vicentini, A. Gropetti, and P. Mantegazza, *Eur. J. Pharmacol*, **36**, 405 (1976).

20. A. H. Abdallah, D. M. Roby, W. H. Boeckler, and C. C. Riley, *Eur. J. Pharmacol.*, **40**, 39 (1976).

21. B. V. Clineschmidt, J. C. McGuffin, and A. B. Werner, *Eur. J. Pharmacol.*, **27**, 313 (1974).

22. R. J. Carey, *Pharmacol. Biochem. Behav.*, **5**, 519 (1976).

23. J. E. Ahlskog, *Brain Res.*, **27**, 211 (1974).

24. R. Samanin, C. Bendotti, S. Bernasconi, E. Borroni, and S. Garattini, *Eur. J. Pharmacol.*, **43**, 117 (1977).

25. F. Borsini, C. Bendotti, M. Carli, E. Poggesi, and R. Samanin, *Res. Commun. Chem. Pathol. Pharmcol.*, **26**, 3 (1979).

26. K. P. Porikos, A. C. Sullivan, B. McGhee and T. B. Van Itallie, *Clin. Pharmacol. Ther.*, **27**, 815 (1980).

27. K. B. J. Franklin and L. J. Herberg, *Neuropharmacol.*, **16**, 45 (1977).

28. A. S. Hollister, G. N. Ervin, B. R. Cooper, and G. R. Breese, *Neuropharmacology*, **14**, 715 (1975).

29. I. S. Sanghvi, G. Singer, E. Friedman, and S. Gershon, *Pharmacol. Biochem. Behav.*, **3**, 81 (1975).

30. S. F. Leibowitz, *Brain Res.*, **98**, 529 (1975).

31. H. Schmitt, *J. Pharmacol.* (Paris), **4**, 285 (1973).

32. Z. L. Kruk, L. A. Smith, and M. R. Zarrindast, *Brit. J. Pharmacol.*, **58**, 468P (1976).

33. J. Duhault, L. Beregi, and F. Roman, *Prog. Neuro-psychopharmacol.*, **4**, 341 (1980).

34. F. Borsini, C. Bendotti, P. Thurlby and R. Samanin, *Life Sci.*, **30**, 905 (1982).

35. R. Samanin, S. Bernasconi, and S. Garattini, *Eur. J. Pharmacol.*, **34**, 373 (1975).

36. T. G. Heffner, M. J. Zigmond, and E. M. Stricker, *J. Pharmacol. Exp. Ther.*, **201**, 386 (1977).

37. S. L. Burridge and J. E. Blundell, *Neuropharmacology*, **18**, 453 (1979).

38. S. Dobrzanski and N. S. Doggett, *Psychopharmacology* (Berlin), **66**, 297 (1979).

39. T. Silverstone, J. Fincham, B. Wells, and M. Kyriakidas, *Neuropharmacology*, **19**, 1235 (1980).

40. M. O. Carruba, S. Ricciardi, E. E. Mueller, and P. Mantegazza, *Eur. J. Pharmacol.*, **64**, 133 (1980).

41. M. O. Carruba, S. Ricciardi, E. E. Mueller, and P. Mantegazza, *Pharmacol. Res. Commun.*, **12**, 599 (1980).

42. J. Vardi, Z. Oberman, I. Rabey, M. Stre'fler, D. Ayalon, and M. Herzberg, *J. Neurol. Sci.*, **30**, 33 (1976).

43. S. F. Liebowitz and C. Rossakis, *Psychopharmacology*, **61**, 273 (1979).

44. R. B. Hemmes, H. M. Pack, and J. Hirsch, *Fed. Proc.*, **38**, 277 (1979).

45. R. B. Hemmes, H. M. Pack, and J. Hirsch, *Fed. Proc.*, **39**, 782 (1980).

46. W. H. Funderburk, J. C. Hazelwood, R. T. Ruckart, and J. W. Ward, *J. Pharm. Pharmacol.*, **23**, 468 (1971).

47. S. Jespersen and J. Scheel-Krüger, *J. Pharm. Pharmacol.*, **25**, 49 (1973).

48. S. Garattini, W. Buczko, A. Jori, and R. Samanin, *Postgrad. Med. J.*, **51**, (Suppl. 1), 27 (1975).

49. A. M. Barrett and L. McSharry, *J. Pharm. Pharmacol.*, **27**, 889 (1975).

50. D. Ghezzi, R. Samanin, S. Bernasconi, G. Tognoni, M. Gerna, and S. Garattini, *Eur. J. Pharmacol.*, **24**, 205 (1973).

51. J. Duhault, M. Boulanger, C. Voisin, C. L. Malen, and H. Schmitt, *Arzneim-Forsch*, **25**, 1758 (1975).

52. B. V. Clineschmidt, *Eur. J. Pharmacol.*, **24**, 405 (1973).

53. M. F. Sugrue, I. Goodlet, and I. McIndewar, *J. Pharm. Pharmacol.*, **27**, 950 (1975).

54. T. B. Wishart and R. M. Zacharko, *Commun. Psychopharmacol.*, **3**, 335 (1979).

55. R. Samanin, T. Mennini, A. Ferraris, C. Bendotti, and F. Borsini, *Eur. J. Pharmacol.*, **61**, 203 (1980).

56. A. C. Sullivan, L. Cheng, and J. G. Hamilton, *Ann. Rep. Med. Chem.*, **11**, 200 (1976).

57. R. Samanin, C. Bendotti, F. Miranda, and S. Garattini, *J. Pharm. Pharmacol.*, **29**, 53 (1977).

58. R. Samanin, C. Bendotti, G. Candelaresi, and S. Garattini, *Life Sci.*, **21**, 1259 (1977).

59. B. V. Clineschmidt, H. M. Hanson, A. B. Flueger, and J. C. McGuffin, *Psychopharmacology*, **55**, 27 (1977).

60. B. V. Clineschmidt, *Gen. Pharmacol.*, **10**, 287 (1979).

61. R. Samanin, T. Mennini, A. Ferraris, C. Bendotti, F. Borsini, and S. Garattini, *Naunyn-Schmiedeberg's Arch. Pharmakol.*, **308**, 159 (1979).

62. R. J. Simpson, D. J. Lawton, M. H. Watt, B. Tiplady, *Brit. J. Clin. Pharmacol.*, **11**, 96 (1981).

63. C. Dumont, J. Laurent, A. Grandadam, and J. R. Boissier, *Life Sci.*, **28**, 1939 (1981).

64. K. Kuriyama and H. Kimura, "Distribution and Possible Functional Roles of GABA in the Retina, Lower Auditory Pathway, and Hypothalamus," in E. Roberts, T. Chase, and D. Tower, Eds., *GABA in Nervous System Function*. Raven, New York, 1976, p. 203.

65. F. Cattabeni, A. Maggi, M. Monduzzi, L. De Angelis, and G. Racagni, *J. Neurochem.*, **31**, 565 (1978).

66. J. Kelly, G. F. Alheid, A. Newberg, and S. P. Grossman, *Pharmacol. Biochem. Behav.*, **7**, 537 (1977).

67. J. Kelly and S. P. Grossman, *Pharmacol. Biochem. Behav.*, **11**, 647 (1979).

68. L. J. Porrino and E. E. Coons, *Pharmacol. Biochem. Behav.*, **12**, 125 (1980).

69. L. Grandison and A. Guidotti, *Neuropharmacology*, **16**, 533 (1977).

70. J. E. Morley and A. S. Levine, *Life Sci.*, **29**, 1213 (1981).

71. B. R. Cooper, J. L. Howard, H. L. White, F. Soroko, K. Ingold, and R. A. Maxwell, *Life Sci.*, **26**, 1997 (1980).

72. J. K. Tews, E. A. Riegel, and A. E. Harper, *Brain Res. Bull.*, **5**, (Suppl. 2), 245 (1980).

73. J. K. Tews, *Life Sci.*, **29**, 2535 (1981).

74. N. Blavet, F. V. DeFeudis, and F. Clostre, *Behav. Neural Biol.*, **34**, 109 (1982).

75. J. L. Howard, H. L. White , B. R. Cooper, and K. W. Rohrbach, *Fed. Proc.*, **41**, 1060 (1982).

76. H. L. White, J. L. Howard, B. R. Cooper, F. E. Soroko, J. D. McDermed, K. J. Ingold, and R. A. Maxwell, *J. Neurochem.*, **39**, 271 (1982).

77. A. C. Sullivan, H. W. Baruth, and L. Cheng, *Ann. Rep. Med. Chem.*, **15**, 172 (1980).

78. P. Turner, *Curr. Med. Res. Opin.*, **6**, (Suppl. 1), 101 (1979).

79. A. C. Sullivan, J. Triscari, and K. Comai, "Antiobesity Agents Acting Through Peripheral Mechanisms," in F. G. De las Heras and S. Vega, Eds., *Seventh International Symposium of Medicinal Chemistry*, Pergamon, Oxford, England, 1981, p. 283.

80. D. N. Brindley and M. Bowley, *Postgrad. Med. J.*, **51**, (Suppl. 1), 91 (1975).

81. M. Ashwell, *J. Clin. Pharmacol.*, **1**, 413 (1974).

82. J. P. Kaye, S. Tomlin, and D. J. Galton, *Postgrad. Med. J.*, **51**, (Suppl. 1), 95 (1975).

83. A. Bizzi, E. Veneroni, and S. Garattini, *Eur. J. Pharmacol.*, **23**, 131 (1973).

84. K. Comai, J. Triscari, and A. C. Sullivan, *Biochem. Pharmacol.*, **27**, 1987 (1978).

85. P. B. Curtis-Prior, A. R. Oblin, and S. Tan, *Int. J. Obes.*, **4**, 111 (1980).

86. W. N. Dannenburg, B. C. Kardian, and L. Y. Norrell, *Arch. Int. Pharmacodyn. Ther.*, **201**, 115 (1973).

87. W. N. Dannenburg and J. W. Ward, *Arch. Int. Pharmacodyn. Ther.*, **191**, 58 (1971).

88. D. Borgström and C. Wollensen, *F.E.B.S. Lett.*, **126**, 25 (1981).

89. T. A. Pasquine and S. W. Thenen, *Proc. Soc. Exp. Biol. Med.*, **166**, 241 (1981).

90. B. Riveline, *Curr. Med. Res. Opin.*, **6**, (Suppl 1), 236 (1979).

91. G. Slama, A. Selmi, M. Hautecouverture, and G. Tchobroutsky, *Diabete Metab.*, **4**, 193 (1978).

92. R. Rath, K. Vondra, A. Bass, V. Kujalova, and J. Wenkeova, *Int. J. Obes.*, **3**, 133 (1979).

93. M. J. Kirby and P. Turner, *Postgrad. Med. J.*, **51**, (Suppl. 1), 73 (1975).

94. M. J. Kirby and P. Turner, *Brit. J. Clin. Pharmacol.*, **1**, 340P (1974).

95. M. J. Kirby, H. Carageorgiou-Markomihalakis, and P. Turner, *Brit. J. Clin. Pharmacol.*, **2**, 541 (1975).

96. M. J. Kirby and P. Turner, *J. Pharm. Pharmacol.*, **28**, 163 (1976).

97. M. J. Kirby and P. Turner, *Brit. J. Clin. Pharmacol.*, **4**, 459 (1977).

98. M. J. Kirby and P. J. Williams, *Abstracts, 7th Int. Congr. Pharm.*, 1978, p. 268.

99. L. C. Harrison, A. P. King-Roach, F. I. R. Martin, and R. A. Melick, *Postgrad. Med. J.*, **51**, (Suppl. 1), 110 (1975).

100. L. C. Harrison and A. P. King-Roach, *Clin. Exp. Pharmacol. Physiol.*, **3**, 503 (1976).

101. J. W. H. Doar, M. E. Thompson, C. E. Wilde, and P. F. J. Sewell, *Curr. Med. Res. Opin.*, **6**, (Suppl. 1), 247 (1979).

102. L. C. Harrison, A. P. King-Roach, and K. C. Sandy, *Metabolism*, **24**, 1353 (1975).

103. A. S. Levine and J. E. Morley, *Science*, **217**, 77 (1982).

104. D. L. Margules, B. Moisset, M. J. Lewis, H. Shibuya, and C. B. Pert, *Science*, **202**, 988 (1978).

105. A. Y. Deutch and R. J. Martin, *Fed. Proc.*, **40**, 905 (1981).

106. L. D. McKay, N. J. Kenney, N. K. Edens, R. H. Williams, and S. C. Woods, *Life Sci.*, **29**, 1429 (1981).

107. J. E. Morley and A. S. Levine, *Life Sci.*, **29**, 1901 (1981).

108. B. Brands, J. A. Thornhill, M. Hirst, and C. W. Gowdey, *Life Sci.*, **24**, 1773 (1979).

109. B. M. King, F. X. Castellanos, A. J. Kastin, M. C. Berzas, M. D. Mauk, R. D. Olson, and G. A. Olson, *Pharmacol. Biochem. Behav.*, **11**, 729 (1979).

110. A. Mandenoff, F. Fumeron, M. Apfelbaum, and D. L. Margules, *Science*, **215**, 1536 (1982).

111. M. T. Lowy, R. P. Maickel and G. K. Yim, *Life Sci.*, **26**, 2113 (1980).

112. R. D. Sewell and K. Jawaharlal, *J. Pharm. Pharmacol.*, **32**, 148 (1980).

113. M. T. Lowy, and G. K. W. Yim, *Life Sci.*, **27**, 2553 (1980).

114. S. M. Antelman and N. Rowland, *Science,* **214,** 1149 (1981).

115. I. M. Lang, J. C. Strahlendorf, H. K. Strahlendorf, and C. D. Barnes, "Effects of Chronic Administration of Naltrexone on Appetitive Behaviors of Rats," in J. B. Lombardini and A. D. Kenny, Eds., *The Role of Peptides and Amino Acids on Neurotransmitters,* Alan R. Liss, New York, 1981, p. 197.

116. M. Kyriakides, T. Silverstone, W. Jeffcoate, and B. Laurance, *Lancet,* **1,** 876 (1980).

117. E. Vijayan and S. M. McCann, *Endocrinology,* **100,** 1727 (1977).

118. R. A. Vogel, B. R. Cooper, T. S. Barlow, A. J. Prange, Jr., R. A. Mueller, and G. R. Bresse, *J. Pharmacol. Exp. Ther.,* **208,** 161 (1979).

119. J. E. Morley and A. S. Levine, *Pharmacol. Biochem. Behav.,* **14,** 149 (1981).

120. J. E. Morley, A. S. Levine, and C. Prasad, *Brain Res.,* **210,** 475 (1981).

121. W. J. Freed, M. J. Perlow, and R. J. Wyatt, *Science,* **206,** 850 (1979).

122. A. S. Levine and J. E. Morley, *Brain Res.,* **222,** 187 (1981).

123. M. J. Perlow, W. J. Freed, J. S. Carman, and R. J. Wyatt, *Pharmacol. Biochem. Behav.,* **12,** 609 (1980).

124. J. Knoll, *Physiol. Behav.,* **23,** 497 (1979).

125. J. Knoll, "Anorectic Agents and Satietin, an Endogenous Inhibitor of Food Intake," in *Proc. 8th Int. Congr. Pharmacol.,* 1981, Vol. 1, 1982, p. 146.

126. J. E. Morley and A. S. Levine, *Eur. J. Pharmacol.,* **67,** 309 (1980).

127. H. Kohno, T. Sakurado, T. Suzuki, K. Kisara, and H. Satoh, *Jpn. J. Pharmacol.,* **31,** 863 (1981).

128. G. P. Smith and J. Gibbs, "Brain-Cut Peptides and the Control of Food Intake," in J. B. Martin, S. Reichlin, and K. L Bick, Eds. *Neurosecretion and Brain Psychopharmacology* (*Advances in Biochemical Psychopharmacology,* Vol. 28). Raven, New York, 1981, p. 389.

129. P. J. Kulkosky, L. Gray, J. Gibbs, and G. P. Smith, *Peptides* (Fayetteville) **4,** Spring, 61 (1981).

130. T. W. Moody, T. L. O'Donohue, and D. M. Jacobowitz, *Peptides,* **2,** 75 (1981).

131. H. R. Kissileff, F. X. Pi-Sunyer, J. Thornton, and G. P. Smith, *Am. J. Clin. Nutr.,* **34,** 154 (1981).

132. G. Statcher, G. Steinringer, G. Schmierer, C. Schneider, and S. Winklehner, *Peptides,* **3,** 133 (1982).

133. F. X. Pi-Sunyer, H. R. Kissileff, J. Thornton, and G. P. Smith, *Am. J. Clin. Nutr.,* **34,** 629 (1981).

134. C. L. McLaughlin and C. A. Baile, *Physiol. Behav.,* **26,** 433 (1981).

135. C. L. McLaughlin and C. A. Baile, *Physiol. Behav.,* **25,** 543 (1980).

136. S. R. Peikin, C. L. McLaughlin, and C. A. Baile, *Fed. Proc.,* **41,** 388 (1982).

137. R. B. Innis, F. M. A. Correa, G. R. Uhl, B. Schneider, and S. H. Snyder, *Proc. Natl. Acad. Sci. U.S.A.,* **76,** 521 (1979).

138. E. Straus and R. S. Yalow, *Science,* **203,** 68 (1979).

139. S. E. Hays and S. M. Paul, *Eur. J. Pharmacol.,* **70,** 591 (1981).

140. J. Hansky and P. Ho, *Aust. J. Exp. Biol. Med. Sci.,* **57,** 575 (1979).

141. B. S. Schneider, J. W. Monahan, and J. Hirsch, *J. Clin. Invest.,* **64,** 1348 (1979).

142. J. A. Finkelstein, A. W. Steggles, F. Lotstra, and J. -J. Vanderhaeghen, *Peptides,* **2,** 19 (1981).

143. J. F. Rehfeld and C. Kruse-Larsen, *Brain Res.,* **155,** 19 (1978).

144. M. A. Della-Fera and C. A. Baile, *Science,* **206,** 471 (1979).

145. M. A. Della-Fera and C. A. Baile, *Physiol. Behav.,* **24,** 943 (1980).

146. M. A. Della-Fera, C. A. Baile, B. S. Schneider, and J. A. Grinker, *Science,* **212,** 687 (1981).

147. M. A. Della-Fera, C. A. Baile, and S. R. Peikin, *Physiol. Behav.,* **26,** 799 (1981).

148. M. L. McCaleb and R. D. Myers, *Peptides* (Fayetteville), **1,** Spring, 47 (1980).

149. C. B. Nemeroff, A. J. Osbahr, III, G. Bissette, G. Jahnke, M. A. Lipton and A. J. Prange, Jr., *Science,* **200,** 793 (1978).

150. J. E. Morley, *Life Sci.,* **30,** 479 (1982).

151. J. N. Hunt, *Am. J. Physiol.,* **239,** G1 (1980).

152. A. C. Sullivan, K. Comai, and J. Triscari "Novel Antiobesity Agents Whose Primary Site of Action is the Gastrointestinal Tract," in P. Bjorntorp, M. Cairella, and A. Howard, Eds., *Recent Advances in Obesity Research, Vol. III,* John Libbey, London, 1981, p. 199.

153. A. C. Sullivan, W. Dairman, and J. Triscari, *Pharmacol. Biochem. Behav.,* **15,** 303 (1981).

154. J. Triscari and A. C. Sullivan, *Pharmacol. Biochem. Behav.,* **15,** 311 (1981).

155. A. C. Sullivan and J. Triscari, "Novel Pharmacological Approaches to the Treatment of Obesity," in G. Bray, Ed., *Recent Advances in Obesity Research, II,* Newman, London, 1978, p. 442.

156. S. N. Sullivan, *Lancet,* **1,** 1140 (1980).

157. M. Feldman, J. H. Walsh, and I. I. Taylor, *Gastroenterology,* **79,** 294 (1980).

158. S. N. Sullivan, L. Lamki, and P. Corcoran, *Lancet,* **11,** 86 (1981).

159. M. R. Rees, R. A. Clark, G. D. Holdsworth, D. C. Barber, and P. J. Howlett, *Brit. J. Clin. Pharmacol.,* **10,** 551 (1980).

160. D. M. Berkowitz and R. W. McCallum, *Clin. Pharmacol. Ther.,* **27,** 414 (1980).

161. E. J. Belair, G. R. Carlson, S. Melamed, J. N. Moss, and M. F. Tansy, *J. Pharm. Sci.,* **70,** 347 (1981).

162. T. H. Moran and P. R. McHugh, *Am. J. Physiol.,* **241,** R25 (1981).

163. T. Yamagishi and H. T. Debas, *Am. J. Physiol.,* 234, E375 (1978).

164. K. A. Houpt and T. R. Houpt, *Physiol. Behav.,* **23,** 925 (1979).

165. C. Scarpignato, G. Zimbara, F. Vitula, and G. Bertaccini, *Arch. Int. Pharmacodyn. Ther.,* **249,** 98 (1981).

166. C. Scarpignato and G. Bertaccini, *Digestion,* **21,** 104 (1981).

167. J. C. Valle-Jones, *Brit. J. Clin. Pract.,* **34,** 72 (1980).

168. Z. Glick, *J. Nutr.,* **111,** 1910 (1981).

169. L. Stein, *Science,* **193,** 46 (1963).

170. D. Lorenz, P. Nardi, and G. P. Smith, *Pharmacol. Biochem. Behav.,* **8,** 405 (1978).

171. M. Webb, N. Bond, and R. Stevens, *Physiol. Behav.,* **14,** 669 (1975).

172. T. L. Powley and C. A. Opsahl, *Am. J. Physiol.,* **226,** 25 (1974).

173. R. G. Carpenter, B. A. Stamoutsos, L. D. Dalton, L. A. Frohman, and S. P. Grossman, *Physiol. Behav.,* **23,** 955 (1979).

174. P. Stark, C. W. Toftz, J. A. Turk, and J. D. Henderson, *Am. J. Physiol.,* **214,** 463 (1968).

175.   T. L. Powley, B. A. MacFarlane, M. S. Markell, and C. A. Opsahl, *Behav. Biol.*, **23,** 306 (1978).

176.   L. Stein and J. Seifter, *Am. J. Physiol.*, **202,** 751 (1962).

177.   S. R. Somner, D. Novin, and M. Le Vine, *Science*, **156,** 983 (1967).

178.   R. Tarrab-Hazdai and H. Edery, *Exp. Neurol.*, **67,** 670 (1980).

179.   L. J. Botticelli and R. J. Wurtman, *Life Sci.*, **24,** 1799 (1979).

180.   K. Jhamandas and M. Sutak, *Br. J. Pharmacol.*, **71,** 201 (1980).

181.   R. T. Bartus, R. L. Dean, III, B. Beer, and A. S. Lippa, *Science*, **217,** 408 (1982).

182.   J. A. Watson, M. Fang, and J. M. Lowenstein, *Arch. Biochem. Biophys.*, **135,** 209 (1969).

183.   J. M. Lowenstein, *J. Biol. Chem.*, **246,** 629 (1971).

184.   A. C. Sullivan, J. G. Hamilton, O. N. Miller, and V. R. Wheatley, *Arch. Biochem. Biophys.*, **150,** 183 (1972).

185.   H. Brunengraber, M. Boutry, and J. M. Lowenstein, *Eur. J. Biochem.*, **82,** 373 (1978).

186.   A. C. Sullivan and J. Triscari, "Possible Interrelationship Between Metabolite Flux and Appetite," in D. Novin, W. Wyrwicka, and G. Bray, Eds., *Hunger: Basic Mechanisms and Clinical Implications*, Raven, New York, 1976, p. 115.

187.   A. C. Sullivan, J. Triscari, J. G. Hamilton, and O. N. Miller, *Lipids*, **9,** 129 (1974).

188.   M. R. C. Greenwood, M. P. Cleary, R. Gruen, D. Blase, J. S. Stern, J. Triscari, and A. C. Sullivan, *Am. J. Physiol.*, **240,** E72 (1981).

189.   A. C. Sullivan and J. Triscari, *Am. J. Clin. Nutr.*, **30,** 767 (1977).

190.   H. Chee, D. R. Romsos, and G. A. Leveille, *J. Nutr.*, **107,** 112 (1977).

191.   E. Panek, G. A. Cook, and N. W. Cornell, *Lipids*, **12,** 814 (1977).

192.   T. Kariya and L. J. Wille, *Biochem. Biophys. Res. Commun.*, **80,** 1022 (1978).

193.   J. Triscari and A. C. Sullivan, *Fed. Proc.*, **40,** 907 (1981).

194.   G. L. S. Pawan, *Proc. Nutr. Soc.*, **33,** 239 (1974).

195.   B. F. Clarke and L. J. P. Duncan, *Lancet*, **1,** 123 (1968).

196.   A. Czyzyk, J. Tawecki, J. Sadowski, I. Ponikowska, and Z. Szczepanik, *Diabetes*, **17,** 492 (1968).

197.   S. Hollobaugh, M. B. Rao, and F. A. Kruger, *Diabetes*, **19,** 45 (1970).

198.   E. Lorch, *Diabetologia*, **7,** 195 (1971).

199.   P. Lefebvre, A. Luyckx, F. Mosora, M. Lacroix, and F. Pirnay, *Diabetologia*, **14,** 39 (1978).

200.   W. J. H. Butterfield and M. J. Wichelow, *Lancet*, **2,** 785 (1968).

201.   K. N. Frayn and P. I. Adnitt, *Biochem. Pharmacol.*, **21,** 3153 (1972).

202.   R. W. Stout, J. D. Brynzell, E. L. Bierman, and D. Porte, Jr., *Diabetes*, **23,** 624 (1974).

203.   F. Meyer, M. Ipabetchi, and H. Clauser, *Nature*, **213,** 203 (1967).

204.   A. Holle, W. Mangels, M. Dreyer, J. Kühnau, and H. Rüdiger, *N. Engl. J. Med.*, **305,** 563 (1981).

205.   P. R. Bratusch-Marrain, A. Korn, Waldhäusl, S. Gasić, P. Nowotny, *Metabolism*, **30,** 946 (1981).

206.   H. Schatz, S. Doci, and R. Höfer, *Diabetologia*, **8,** 1 (1972).

207.   M. Cigolini, O. Bosello, A. Bataggia, F. Ferrari, S. Montresor, L. A. Scuro, and U. Smith, *Diabetologia*, **21,** 260 (1981).

208. D. Luft, R. M. Schmülling, and M. Eggstein, *Diabetologia*, **14**, 75 (1978).

209. University Group Diabetes Program, *Diabetes*, **24**, (Suppl. 1), 65 (1975).

210. H. Keen, *J. Clin. Path.*, **28**, (Suppl. 9), 99 (1975).

211. D. D. Schmidt, W. Frommer, B. Junge, L. Müller, W. Wingender, and E. Truscheit, *Naturwissenschaften*, **64**, 535 (1977).

212. W. Puls, U. Keup, H. P. Krause, G. Thomas, and F. Hoffmeister, *Naturwissenschaften*, **64**, 536 (1977).

213. R. H. Taylor, D. J. A. Jenkins, and R. Nineham, *Gut*, **19**, A969 (1978).

214. J. C. McLoughlin and K. D. Buchanan, *Lancet*, **2**, 603 (1979)

215. H. Laube, M. Fouladfar, R. Aubell, and H. Schmitz, *Arzneim.-Forsch*, **30**, 1154 (1980).

216. W. Puls and H. P. Krause, "Delay of Carbohydrate Absorption by Inhibitors of Intestinal α-Glucosidases," in R. A. Cameridinidavalos and B. Hanover, Eds., *Treatment of Early Diabetes* (*Advances in Experimental Medicine and Biology*, Vol. 119), Plenum, New York, 1979, p. 341.

217. R. S. Gray and J. M. Olefsky, *Metab. Clin. Exp.*, **31**, 88 (1982).

218. I. Zavaroni and G. M. Reaven, *Metabolism*, **30**, 417 (1981).

219. H. P. Krause, U. Keup, G. Thomas, and W. Puls, *Metabolism*, **31**, 710 (1982).

220. Z. Glick and G. A. Bray, *Fed. Proc.*, **40**, 916 (1981).

221. E. Haraczkiewicz and J. R. Vasselli, *Fed. Proc.*, **10**, 916 (1981).

222. W. Pirson and P. Buchschacher, *Diabetologia*, **21**, 315 (1981).

223. J. E. Blundell, E. Tombros, P. J. Rogers, and C. J. Latham, *Prog. Neuropsychopharmacol.*, **4**, 319 (1980).

224. J. E. Blundell and C. J. Latham, *Pharmacol. Biochem. Behav.*, **12**, 717 (1980).

225. S. J. Cooper and K. F. Sweeney, *Neuropharmacology*, **19**, 997 (1980).

226. P. J. Rogers and J. E. Blundell, *Psychopharmacology* (Berlin), **66**, 159 (1979).

227. M. Kyriakides and T. Silverstone, *Neuropharmacology*, **18**, 1007 (1979).

228. S. Hsiao, C. H. Wang, and T. Schallert, *Physiol. Behav.*, **23**, 909 (1979).

229. A. J. Strohmayer and G. P. Smith, *Peptides* (Fayetteville), **2**, Spring, 39 (1981).

230. J. A. Grinker, A. Drewnowski, and A. C. Sullivan, *Fed. Proc.*, **41**, 338 (1982).

231. J. J. Wurtman and R. J. Wurtman, *Curr. Med. Res. Opin.*, **6**, (Suppl. 1), 28 (1979).

232. J. J. Wurtman, "Neurotransmitter Regulation of Protein and Carbohydrate Consumption," in S. A. Miller, Ed., *Nutrition and Behavior*, Franklin Institute Press, 1981, p. 69.

233. J. J. Wurtman and R. J. Wurtman, *Am. J. Clin. Nutr.*, **34**, 651 (1981).

234. R. B. Kanarek, L. Ho, and R. G. Meade, *Pharmacol. Biochem. Behav.*, **14**, 539 (1981).

235. A. J. Stunkard, "Anorectic Agents: A Theory of Action and Lack of Tolerance in a Clinical Trial," in S. Garattini and R. Samanin, Eds., *Anorectic Agents: Mechanisms of Action and Tolerance*, Raven, New York, 1981, p. 191.

11

Drugs and Diet Therapy

ALBERT STUNKARD, M.D.

University of Pennsylvania, Philadelphia, Pennsylvania

Let us begin this chapter with a discussion of the drugs that we currently use for the treatment of obesity—the phenfluoramines—which act on the central nervous system. First, these drugs perhaps should be used in the treatment of obesity either indefinitely for very long periods or not at all. We recommend this because they act, I believe, by lowering the body weight set point, they do not rapidly lose their efficacy, at least in humans, tolerance does not develop, and therefore, when they are withdrawn, the body weight set point that had been artificially suppressed by the drug is elevated to the pretreatment level, resulting in very severe pressures upon people to regain the weight they lost with the aid of these drugs. We were alerted to this problem and devised this theory to account for the results of a large-scale clinical trial that was designed to look at the relative efficacy of behavior therapy and of drug therapy in the treatment of obesity.

It is interesting that these two probably most common forms of treatment of obesity, behavior therapy and drug therapy, at least in the treatment of mild obesity have grown up in almost complete isolation. There have been at least 100 well-controlled clinical trials of behavior therapy and there have been hundreds of trials of drug therapy, but until this study, there has been no attempt to compare their relative efficacy by treating patients within the same experimental design, and that is what we tried to do in our study.

In a large-scale study we looked at behavior therapy conducted in groups, as it usually is, and at medication, which was also administered in groups with a sort of placebo talking therapy, and then we looked at the combination with fairly large numbers of patients. These patients were all women who were 65% overweight, middle aged, middle class, and the usual kind of patient who comes for treatment of mild moderate obesity.

169

We divided them into booster and no booster sessions to try to determine a method of improving the maintenance of weight lost in the treatment of obesity by having sessions with decreasing frequency, so that during the treatment periods all patients are treated once a week and then afterwards in the booster group every two weeks and then every month and then every two months. The no booster group was cut off after the initial treatment period.

In addition we had two control groups. One was a waiting list group—the no treatment control in which we told patients we would treat them after a while but that the treatment groups were filled. The second was a doctor's office medication group in which we had general practice residents play the part of the friendly family doctor who worked on a protocol that involved getting the patients in, working them up, getting histories, doing physical examinations, telling them they were too fat, telling them they had to lose weight, giving them a diet, and giving them the drug that we used in this study, phenfluoramine. They then followed the patients every few weeks. They carried out the usual medical therapy to compare this with the other two groups.

At the end of six months of treatment the waiting list control group gained weight, the doctor's office medication group lost about 13 pounds, the behavior modification group lost about 23 pounds, and the group that received placebo but approximately the same amount of attention that the behavior modification people got lost 30–31 pounds. Based on these results we combined the two with the idea that maybe we could get the best of both forms of treatment. We would get all this fine magic that is involved in behavior modification and then speed up weight loss with a drug. However, we found that we did not speed up weight loss. Combining the two treatments did not increase the rate at which people lost weight. At this point we thought that maybe the answer to the treatment of obesity is simply to use phenfluoramine and not worry about this slower, less effective kind of treatment, behavior modification. We thought that it would be interesting to see what happened over a period of time, and so we followed these patients—a very large number of patients—and were able to follow up every patient in the study. Over one hundred patients were followed up a year later, and revealed very striking differences. At the end of the year patients in the behavior modification group were still about 8 kg below their pretreatment weight. By contrast, the pharmotherapy group rebounded rather rapidly, so that although they had lost significantly more weight at the end of treatment, a year later they weighed significantly more. That result was not unexpected, since it has been found in many patients and in animal studies. What was really striking was the result of combined treatment. We had reasoned that maybe combining treatments would allow us to take advantage of the rapid weight loss with the drug and then to teach the patient behavioral techniques that would enable them to keep the weight off. In fact, they did almost statistically significantly worse than the people who had drug treatment alone; it looked almost as if the addition of the drug to the behavioral treatment had compromised its effectiveness in maintenance of weight loss.

Two or three of the conclusions we drew from this study run somewhat in the face of traditional views about the use of drugs. One has to do with the issue of tolerance. It looked to us from three points of view as though tolerance had not developed to the effects of phenfluoramine over the period of as long as six months, which is a good long period in the usual clinical trial, and the three forms of evidence are first that the slowing of weight loss was occurring less in the drug-treated group than in the behavior modification group and actually not slowing very much even at the end of six months. Part of that slowing was because some of the patients were reaching their normal weights and so could not lose any more weight. Hence by that one criterion—slowing of weight loss—tolerance had not developed. Now that is not a particularly sensitive measure but at least it is one measure. The second criterion was that we had measures of hunger during this period and what one would expect if tolerance had developed to the effects of this drug is that hunger would increase. However, over the six months of this treatment hunger slightly decreased in patients on phenfluoramine, suggesting that there was no breakthrough of the loss of effectiveness of the drug. Finally, this very rapid rebound would suggest that the drug was still active and that when it was withdrawn people were responding by rapid weight gain. The most ready explanation of these findings to us was that the drug worked by lowering the body weight set point, lowering the regulatory level, and that when the drug was withdrawn that set point bounced back up to the pretreatment level, causing very strong biological pressures on the person to regain the weight. We have since repeated this study and found the same results. Let us now examine some evidence from the animal literature that would support this.

The evidence has to do with the idea that body weight is regulated. It is not immediately apparent that body weight is regulated, particularly in fat people and animals. In fact, some years ago it was thought that obesity was due to a breakdown in the regulation because why would animals and people be fat if they were regulating their body weight appropriately? The first evidence against this was obtained by Hovel and Teitelbaum some years ago when they looked at the regulation of animals made obese by lesions in the ventromedial hypothalamus. The way of finding out whether regulation occurs is to perturb the system and see what happens when you remove the perturbation. For example, in normal weight animals or normal weight people, if you starve them and then let them eat again their body weight will come back to what it had been. If you overfeed them by a variety of methods, get them fat and then let them eat normally, body weight comes back down to the pretreatment level. What Hovel and Teitelbaum did was to take rats made fat by ventromedial lesions and apply the same kind of tests, and they found that these rats actually did regulate body weight. If the fat rat were made even fatter by tube feeding or by giving him insulin injections or through various other methods and if then those interventions were removed, his body weight would come back to normal. So the question is, if these fat rats regulate so well why are they fat? And the argument was made that they are fat because the lesions resulted in an elevation of a body weight set point. According to the thinking at the time, the ventromedial hypothalamus was functioning as a kind of brake on appetite and on eating, and if you destroyed that the animal should go out and eat more. So they raised the body weight of these rats and then put in the lesion. The question was, did they become obese because they overeat to become obese? They showed that a rat made obese by insulin injection and then given the lesion maintains body weight at the same level. When he is starved, he loses weight, and when he is allowed to eat again he regains it. It looks, therefore, as if by raising the weight to the level that would be reached as a result of the lesion one can prevent the lesion from having any special effect upon the body weight. This is interpreted as evidence that the lesion is acting by elevating the body weight set point. Now there is a kind of symmetrical series of observations on lowering of body weight by lateral hypothalamic lesions. These animals also appear to regulate their body weight. Thin animals made thin by lesions in the lateral hypothalamus undereat for a period of time but then their weight slowly increases. If you take one of them out and overfeed him with a tube feeding and then remove the tube feeding and allow him to eat ad lib, his body weight will come back down, and similarly if you starve these animals they lose weight just as the control animals do and then when they are allowed to eat freely again they overeat until their body weight comes back to the previous level just as the normal animals do. So it looks as if these thin animals are also regulating body weight. The question is, are they thin because of a lowered body weight set point? Dr. Kesey did a study similar to the one mentioned before with the obesity and that was to lower body weight to the level that it would be expected to reach with a lateral hypothalamic lesion and then see if the lesion further lowered body weight. What Kesey did in this study was to lower the body weight before the lesion, and then put in the lesion. What happened was that following the lesion, which up until this time absolutely predictably lowered body weight, body weight increased. It is a striking phenomenon, suggesting that the effect of the lesion is determined by the body weight at the time the lesion is made. Now it seemed to me when I saw this work that this would be a perfect model for a pharmacological study to see if a drug would have this same effect. In other words, if you lowered body weight of an animal and then gave it a drug, could you get it to overeat even in the face of an appetite suppressant, if the body weight of the animal were below this putative set point? And, last summer a paper appeared by David Levitsky at Cornell University showing exactly this, and this is a somewhat oversimplified version of David Levitsky's study. He had a normal control group and a group that was given drugs, and he did this with both phenfluoramine and amphetamine, so that although the clinical findings apply only to phenfluoramine this looks as if it would also happen with amphetamine and so might be extended to all of the drugs working through central nervous system action.

What happens is that the animal loses weight and then seems to regulate at a lower level very much as the animals who receive the lateral hypothalamic lesions do. Then, when the drug is withdrawn, he regains weight back to normal. Now the critical experiment was to lower the body weight before giving the drug, and it was found that if you lower the body weight before giving the drug and then give this drug that should suppress appetite, you see a very rapid weight gain—increased eating until the body weight gets back to the level of the animal that never had it reduced but received drugs—and then they continue on regulating rather well until the drug is removed and then body weight goes back up to normal. The best interpretation of these results, although I don't think Levitsky would interpret them this way, is that the drug is lowering the body weight set point and that removal of the drug raises the set point back to its previous level. In fact, there are three other studies in the literature that suggest the very same thing, although the authors of these studies have not interpreted the results this way.

I would like to close by discussing very briefly the clinical implications of these findings. The fact that tolerance apparently does not develop to the effect of phenfluoramine means that the old argument against its use—that is, loss of efficacy and development of tolerance, is no longer valid. Phenfluoramine appears to retain its efficacy and paradoxically this fact provides a new argument against current recommendations that it be used only for short periods of time. For if the medication lowers the body weight set point, discontinuing its use with elevation of the set point to its previous level may compromise the ability of an obese person to maintain weight losses achieved with the help of the medication. If phenfluoramine and possibly other medications are to be useful at all, perhaps they should be used only for very long periods of time. These facts and this theory suggest that we need to reevaluate our current practices in drug therapy for obesity.

12

Diuretics and Salt Restriction in Blood Pressure Control

SYLVIA WASSERTHEIL-SMOLLER, Ph.D.

Albert Einstein College of Medicine, Bronx, New York,

HERBERT G. LANGFORD, M.D.

University of Mississippi, Jackson, Mississippi

M. DONALD BLAUFOX, M.D., Ph.D.

Albert Einstein College of Medicine, Bronx, New York

ALBERT OBERMAN, M.D.

University of Alabama in Birmingham, Birmingham, Alabama

MORT HAWKINS, Sc.D.

University of Texas, Houston, Texas

Many remedies have been tried for hypertension control which, with time, have proved to be of little value (1). Now it seems that everyone has rediscovered low-salt therapy. Virtually all the official guidelines and most physicians recommend that hypertensive patients reduce their salt

Supported by NHLBI.

intake, as if it were a new treatment and as if its efficacy were proven. Neither is true. It is not a new discovery and it is not yet scientifically established that salt restriction, or what degree of it, can control high blood pressure, although there are studies in progress addressing these issues and these will be discussed.

Low-salt diets were advocated as early as 1904 in France (2) and 1922 in the United States (3), but perhaps the most famous is the Kempner Rice-Fruit Diet (4). This diet was described in 1948 and consists of 2000 calories a day and 150 mg of sodium, or about 7 meq. Kempner reported that of 500 patients treated, 62% improved. It also was a weight reduction regimen and a high-potassium diet. It is not clear which of these has the most beneficial effect on blood pressure. This was not a clinical trial and was hardly definitive. In any case, in the 1950s there was a rapid development of antihypertensive drugs and attention was drawn to pharmacological agents.

The first well-controlled, double-blind placebo trial of drug therapy for hypertension conducted by the Veterans Administration (5, 6) clearly demonstrated the beneficial effect on morbidity and mortality of pharmacologically treating high blood pressure for moderate and severe hypertensives (i.e., those with diastolic blood pressure greater than 105 mm Hg), but it left unanswered the question of what to do with the mild hypertensives (those with diastolic pressures of 90–104 mm Hg) and whether this beneficial effect would extend to women, to younger individuals, and to blacks.

To answer some of these questions, the Hypertension Detection and Follow-Up Program (HDFP) was mounted by the National Heart, Lung, and Blood Institute in the early 1970s (7, 8). The HDFP was a 17-center collaborative trial which studied over 10,000 hypertensive patients and followed them for five years. They were divided by random assignment into stepped and referred care groups. Stepped care participants were treated in specially set up HDFP clinics with a stepped protocol, beginning with diuretics and adding drugs successively for patients who had not reached goal blood pressure. Goal blood pressure was a diastolic pressure of 90 mm Hg for participants with entry pressures of 100 mm Hg or above, or already receiving antihypertensive therapy and it was a 10 mm decrease for participants whose entry pressure were between 90 and 99 mm Hg. The stepped care regimen is shown in Table 1. At the end of one year, 39% had attained the goal blood pressure with diuretics alone and another 24% with diuretics plus either reserpine or methyldopa (9, 10). The other half of the hypertensives were assigned to referred care, meaning that they would be treated by their usual sources of care—private physicians or other community sources of care.

Table 1.   Stepped Care Treatment Schedule

Step No.	Drug(s) Used	Dose (mg/day)	Duration (Max.)
0	None	—	—
1	Chlorthalidone	25–100	4 wks for dosage
	or		
	spironolactone	25–100	12 wks for step
2	Add reserpine	0.1–0.25	4 to 12 weeks
	or		
	methyldopa	500–2000	4 to 12 wks
3	Add hydralazine	30–200	4 to 16 wks
4	Add quanethidine	10–200	Open
5	Other drugs as indicated	—	—

The basic results of the HDFP are shown in Figure 1 indicating that intensive stepped care pharmacologic treatment of hypertensive patients resulted in a 17% decrease in mortality when compared to a group of patients whose blood pressure was being managed by their usual sources of medical care (11, 12). Of particular importance is the finding that the *mild* hypertensives showed a 20% reduction in mortality in the stepped care group compared to the referred care group. It is worthwhile to note

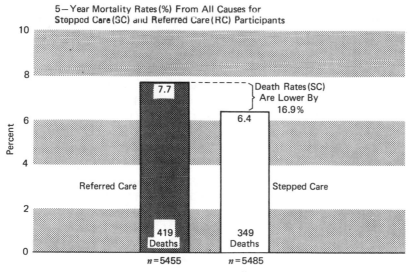

Figure 1.   Mortality, all causes.

that about 70% of hypertensives are in the "mild hypertension" category, i.e., having diastolic blood pressure between 90 and 104 mm Hg. This represents approximately 25 million people in the United States. The issue of whether these people should be subjected to a lifetime of drugs for hypertension is an important one both in terms of potential long-term side effects, the unpleasantness of lifetime drug therapy, and the extensive health care cost implied by such a public policy. Thus, there is a renewed interest in the possibility of the control of blood pressure through nonpharmacologic means, such as weight reduction and salt restriction.

Several major questions arise about salt restriction. First, will salt restriction *prevent* hypertension? This question is being addressed by a recently begun trial of the Primary Prevention of Hypertension led by the Birmingham, Alabama, group which is attempting to determine whether individuals with normal blood pressures can be prevented from developing elevations of blood pressure through salt restriction. Second, will salt restriction *control* hypertension? This question is being addressed by a study to be discussed below: the Dietary Intervention Study of Hypertension. And, third, is it *feasible* to reduce salt intake to an effective level? How low must salt intake be in order to be effective? Sir George Pickering, for example, described as one of the major limitations of the Kempner diet "the extent to which it disrupts social relations." Dr. Pickering said, "it is insipid, unappetizing, and monotonous and demands great care of its preparation for if salt rises above 250 mg the effect in most instances is lost. In Great Britain, it is quite impracticable for a member of a large household with minimum domestic help. In the United States, where salt-free articles are more easily obtained from stores, it becomes a practical proposition. Even then, its deadly monotony tends to make it intolerable unless the physician can infuse into the patient some of the aceticism of the religious zealot. In using this diet, it is essential to check the urinary excretion of sodium or chloride, which should not exceed 5 meq of sodium per day" (13).

This obviously is an extremely rigorous diet. The Dietary Intervention Study of Hypertension (DISH) addresses the question whether *modest* restriction in sodium can control blood pressure. The patient population comes from the Hypertension Detection and Follow-Up Program. Of the 17 centers that were participants in the HDFP, four centers are participating in the new DISH trial: three clinical centers at Jackson, Mississippi; Birmingham, Alabama; and New York, New York, and a Computer Coordinating Center at Houston, Texas. The 590 DISH participants are individuals whose blood pressure was previously controlled to be below 90 mm Hg with drugs in the HDFP. The primary objective of DISH is to determine whether weight reduction or sodium restriction can maintain blood pressure control without the use of antihypertensive drugs. The goal electrolyte intake for the salt restriction participants is 70 meq or 1.6 g. We are interested in seeing: (1) whether it is feasible to get individuals to reduce their intake to 70 meq, and (2) whether this relatively modest reduction is sufficient to control previously drug-controlled hypertensives.

The design of DISH (Figure 2) shows the randomization of patients into seven groups, stratified by obesity. Patients who are above 120% ideal weight are randomly assigned into one of four groups: (1) those who are to continue medication as in the HDFP, (2) those who are to be withdrawn from medication over a period of time and who will receive no intervention, (3) those who are to be discontinued from medication and are in an intervention group with the objective of restricting sodium and increasing potassium, and (4) those who are withdrawn from medication and in the intervention group for weight reduction. The nonobese individuals, those whose weight is less than or equal to 120% ideal weight, are randomly assigned into (5) a group who are to continue medication, or (6) a group who are to discontinue medication with no intervention, or (7) those whose medication is discontinued and who are in the sodium restriction intervention group. The number of subjects randomized to each of these groups is shown below the boxes. This paper will primarily discuss those who are randomized into the salt restriction groups.

All patients entering the study had diastolic blood pressures of 90 mm Hg or less, on pharmacologic treatment. In patients who are withdrawn from hypertensive medication, blood pressure is followed closely and drug therapy is reinstituted if the pressure rises above specific and rather complicated sequential cut points. Individuals who are reinstituted into drug therapy are considered "treatment failures."

An important feature of all such studies is the ability to estimate sodium intake in individuals. There are essentially two ways to estimate

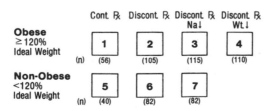

Figure 2.   Dish randomization.

such intake: one is through analysis of food intake by portion analysis or food record analysis, and the other is through analysis of urinary sodium excretion. Although urinary excretion has generally been regarded as a more accurate estimate than food record analysis, urinary excretion itself is highly variable and the practical aspect of 24-hour urine collection may pose inordinate problems, potentially resulting in poor collections and thus poor estimates. In our study, we use both methods of estimation. Initially, patients are assembled for a group session where the program is explained, informed consent is obtained, and instructions are given for keeping a three-day food record and for collecting a 24-hour urine. At the DISH baseline clinic visit, one week following the group meeting, participants bring the three-day food record and 24-hour urine collection to the clinic. The nutritionist reviews the three-day food record individually with each participant. Blood pressures, weights, and heights are recorded, and blood chemistries are performed; histories are taken and physical examinations given. At this time, participants are told whether or not they are in an intervention group. For those randomized to intervention groups, appointments are made for group meetings, which are scheduled every week for eight weeks, and after that individual meetings with the nutritionist are instituted for dietary maintenance.

The dietary and urinary data are collected at baseline, at the clinic revisit which occurs after the eight weeks of dietary intervention, and at the 32 and 56 week visits. Urine collection is started on the day prior to the clinic visit and coincides exactly with the third day of the three-day food record. The food records are analyzed by our Computer Nutrient Analysis System, which analyzes the nutrient content of dietary histories through a descriptive listing of food items and quantities provided by the patient. The food items are coded by a trained and certified staff of coders, keypunched, and then processed in the New York center through the Albert Einstein College of Medicine computer system. The Computer Nutrient Analysis System provides 71 nutrient components of the food records. While our primary interest is in sodium and potassium as well as calories, we have looked at a variety of other nutrients to see whether there are any changes in dietary patterns as a result of the intervention.

Figure 3 shows the baseline data of sodium intake as estimated by urinary and dietary measures at the three different centers. The scale on the left gives the values in milliequivalents and the scale on the right provides the values in milligrams. In Birmingham, the urinary sodium output at baseline was 157 meq or 3611 mg. The dietary estimate was 123 meq or 2829 mg. The caloric average intake was reported to be 1711 calories. The Jackson, Mississippi, center had a slightly lower urinary

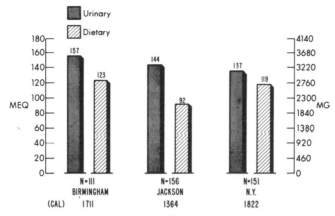

Figure 3. Sodium by center.

output estimate and a considerably lower dietary sodium intake estimate. The reason for this is that the Jackson center had many regional foods that were not included in the computer data base. We have since had them analyzed and the relationship between dietary and urinary estimates is expected to be better in this center.

Figure 4 shows the potassium intake at baseline by center. It is interesting to note, first, that the urinary and dietary potassium estimates are extremely close and, second, that potassium intake was the highest in the New York center and the lowest in the Jackson center. All participants in Jackson are black and 70% of participants in New York are white.

It is methodologically of interest to note to what extent dietary estimates of sodium intake under- or overestimate urinary estimates. Table 2 shows the relationship between dietary and urinary calculations by

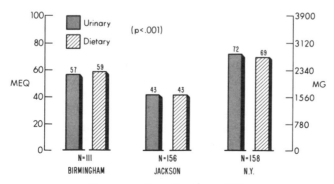

Figure 4. Potassium by center.

Table 2. Dietary Sodium as % of Urinary by Race, Sex, Weight

	(N)	Av D/U (%)	(1 − D/U) %
All	(418)	86.3	9.9
Race = white	(144)	105.9	−5.8
Race = black	(274)	79.7	18.1
Sex = male	(168)	91.6	8.5
Sex = female	(250)	80.6	10.8
Obese			
> 120% Ideal weight	(283)	83.6	16.4
Nonobese			
≤ 120% Ideal weight	(135)	103.9	−3.9

race, sex, and obesity. The averages for 418 individuals studied at baseline showed that the dietary estimate of sodium intake was 86.3% of the urinary estimate, that is, dietary records underestimated urinary sodium by 9.9%, on the average. For whites, however, the dietary estimate was 105.9% of the urinary, representing a 5.9% overestimate, while for blacks, dietary records had an average of 18.1% underestimate. There was no difference between sexes; however, obese individuals tended to underestimate their urinary sodium by about 16.4% while the nonobese individuals overestimated it by 3.9%. Since the sodium intake is related to calories, it is possible that obese individuals underestimate their caloric intake when they keep dietary records.

Now let us see what we were able to accomplish after the intervention for sodium restriction. Figure 5 shows the urinary output for the groups randomized to drug withdrawal and sodium restriction intervention at baseline and at eight weeks after intervention. It can be seen that for the 87 participants randomized to sodium restriction who completed at least eight weeks in the study, there has been a substantial reduction in sodium intake, from 157 meq at baseline to 93 meq at eight weeks. This reduction appears to have been maintained 32 weeks after enrollment into the study. An interesting observation is that the older individuals, those over age 60, were able to reduce their sodium intake to a greater extent than the younger ones, that is, those under 60. The older individuals went from an initially higher sodium output of 175 meq (4025 mg) to 84 meq (1932 mg), while the younger ones started out with a lower output of 144 meq (3312 mg) and got down to 99 meq (2227 mg) after eight weeks. Note, however, that the sodium output of 93 meq (2139 mg) is still substantially above our goal of 70 meq (1610 mg). We were

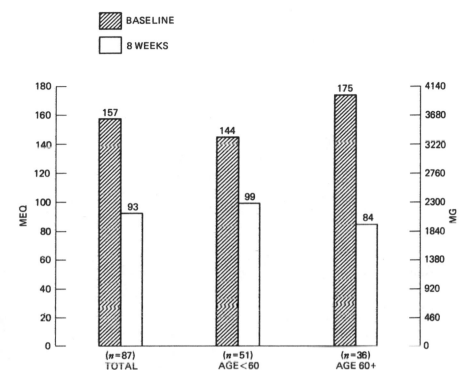

Figure 5.   Urinary output for sodium restriction, drug withdrawal groups.

not able to get our participants to reduce their sodium intake to as low a level as we had initially intended.

The question arose whether we were doing better in reducing sodium intake in those with mild hypertension than in those with more severe levels of blood pressure elevation. Figure 6 shows that for those individuals who started out in the original Hypertension Detection and Follow-Up Program about seven years ago with diastolic blood pressures of 90–104 mm Hg, there was a reduction from 147 to 87 meq of sodium after eight weeks, whereas for those who initially had blood pressure elevations of 105 or more, there was a reduction from 152 to 95 meq, not much difference. Hence, it appears that the initial blood pressure level did not have an effect on the sodium reduction potential of these individuals.

We had hoped to be able to raise the potassium intake of our participants, but in fact we were not really able to do this to any substantial degree, partially because some of our participants were on potassium sup-

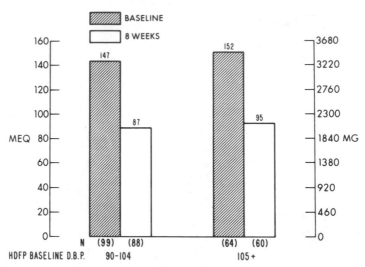

Figure 6. Urinary sodium output by HDFP baseline diastolic blood pressure.

plements at baseline and these were withdrawn along with the antihypertensive drugs. The sodium : potassium ratio showed a decline from 3.3 at baseline to 2.4 after eight weeks of intervention. This decline in the sodium : potassium ratio is attributed to a decline in the sodium rather than to an increase in the potassium.

We said before that sodium was highly related to caloric intake and the question is whether we were able to change the eating patterns of the individuals in the sodium intervention group. We measure that by computing the sodium per calorie at baseline and at eight weeks. Table 3 shows that for the control group with no dietary intervention, the sodium per calorie ratio remained the same; in the weight reduction group it increased, though not significantly, and in the sodium restriction group it declined significantly. Thus, we were able to accomplish a sig-

Table 3. Sodium/Calorie (mg)

Randomization Group	n	Baseline (Mean)	8-Week (Mean)
Control	120	1.56	1.54
Weight reduction	49	1.54	1.70
Sodium restriction	89	1.52	.92[a]

[a] $p < .001$.

nificant change in eating patterns in the sodium restriction group with respect to sodium intake.

Did we also change other nutrients? Table 4 shows that the intakes of a variety of vitamins and minerals were relatively unchanged after eight weeks. Calories went down slightly, but this was not a significant difference. However, total fat and total saturated fat were significantly reduced at eight weeks for the sodium restriction group, accounting for the lower calories noted.

Thus, we have shown that it is possible to reduce sodium intake to approximately 90 meq in a free-living hypertensive population without terribly much difficulty. In fact, some individuals were able to lower sodium substantially. While at baseline about 10% of individuals had a urinary sodium output of 60 meq or less (i.e., 1380 mg) after eight weeks, 42% had this low an output. At baseline 35% had outputs of 180 meq (4140 mg) or more whereas eight weeks later only 7% had such high outputs.

The question then is does this reduced sodium intake control blood pressure without drugs? We cannot answer yet because the study has not

Table 4.   Sodium Restriction Drug Withdrawal Groups ($n = 90$)

RDA	Selected Nutrients	Baseline (Mean)	8-Week (Mean)
—	Fiber (gm)	3.90	4.31
6.0	Ascorbic acid (mg)	136	146
1.0–1.2	Thiamin (B_1) (mg)	1.21	1.05
13–18	Niacin (mg)	18.4	18.0
1.2–1.4	Riboflavin (B_2) (mg)	1.39	1.25
3.0	B_{12} (μg)	4.50	3.58
4000–5000	Vitamin A (IU)	7356	7698
200	Vitamin D (IU)	39.2	29.6
—	Caffeine (mg)	213	226
10–18	Iron (mg)	13.0	11.9
800	Calcium (mg)	546	507
	Calories	1713	1569
	Cholesterol (mg)	326	308
	Total fat (gm)	74	61[a]
	Total saturated fat (gm)	22	18[b]
	Total polyunsaturated fat (gm)	12	10
	Alcohol (gm)	5.4	4.5
	Magnesium (mg)	172	155

[a] $p < .025$.
[b] $p < .01$.

been completed. A variety of earlier studies have been done, however, most of which seem to indicate that there is some blood pressure response to modest levels of sodium restriction (14–16). These studies have generally been on quite small numbers of subjects, ranging from about 17 to 40. The DISH study differs in that it is quite large; there are 197 subjects in the sodium restriction groups and 187 in the control groups. Its objective is to see whether previously drug-controlled hypertensives can maintain this control with salt restriction alone, for which it is more difficult to get compliance than for drug taking. It is clear that there are many other issues that we need to examine carefully. For example, we need to look at the subgroup of individuals who achieved the reduction in sodium that was initially designed, we need to focus on the sodium : potassium ratio and look at the failure rate in relation to that, and we need to see what happens after a longer time of follow-up. It is expected that each patient in this study will have at least 56 weeks of follow-up.

Another important question is whether sodium restriction can decrease the dosage of drugs necessary to control hypertension. Preliminary results indicate that this may indeed be possible. If so, that would support the hypothesis that sodium-depleted individuals have an increased salt appetite, therefore consume more salt, and the increased sodium intake counteracts the effects of the diuretic therapy which results in the salt depletion.

Work by Dr. Herbert Langford and colleagues showed that in 27 black women on antihypertensive therapy including a diuretic, sodium excretion was significantly higher than in 171 women who were on no antihypertensive therapy. Those patients with a diastolic pressure less than or equal to 100 mm Hg receiving treatment excreted 221 meq of sodium per 24 hours, while those not receiving treatment excreted 122.4 meq of sodium per 24 hours. These investigators also reported that the salt taste threshold in 67 patients before, and from two to four weeks after, the institution of diuretic therapy dropped significantly. Dr. Langford comments that these studies suggest that "diuretic induced sodium deprivation in man and rat is associated with increased salt ingestion and with a decreased salt taste threshold which may be part of the mechanism signalling an increased salt appetite" (17).

The highlights of our findings in the DISH study so far are the following:

1. The decrease in urinary sodium output after eight weeks of intervention was about 60 meq or 1380 mg.

2. We have not been able to achieve a mean sodium output of 70 meq. The average attained was about 90 meq or 2070 mg, although a substantial proportion of patients did achieve an intake corresponding to less than 70 meq.

3. We have not increased the potassium output in the sodium restriction group.

4. There is a suggestion, not confirmed because of still small numbers, that blacks were able to lower their sodium to a greater degree than whites after the eight-week intervention period but may not have been as easily able to keep it down as the whites.

5. Urinary sodium went down by a substantially greater amount in individuals 60 years old and over than among those under age 60 in the sodium intervention groups. Urinary potassium also went down substantially in the older groups.

6. Dietary estimates of sodium intake can be very close to 24-hour urinary estimates of sodium output and are sometimes more practical to obtain.

7. Obese individuals tend to give dietary histories that underestimate their urinary sodium output by about 16%, whereas the nonobese overestimate by about 4%.

In summary, the question of salt restriction and its efficacy in controlling high blood pressure is not yet completely resolved. We hope to provide some answers toward its resolution. There are, in fact, two issues: the issue of individual patient therapy and the issue of public health policy. With respect to individual patient therapy, it will be important to identify those individuals who are salt sensitive, to develop cost effective means for implementing intervention programs if such intervention turns out to be a substitute for drug control, and to further study the effect of the sodium : potassium ratio.

With respect to public policy, the question is whether or not lower salt content of foods should be advocated for the general public. This issue would be particularly important if it could be shown that a low salt intake prevents the development of hypertension. The incidence of hypertension in this country is very high and prevalence is about 40% among blacks and about 19% among whites (18). Thus, preventing the development of high blood pressure would be a very important public health measure. The issue of whether salt restriction is effective in *primary prevention* is currently being addressed in the collaborative Primary Prevention of Hypertension Trial, whose objective is to determine whether normotensive individuals who are at higher risk for developing hypertension by virtue of family history can be prevented from such progression of blood pressure elevation by modest sodium restriction. This study, led by the Birmingham, Alabama, center, has just begun and the results will not be in for another five years or so.

The question, of course, is "what to do until the revolution comes," that is, what are we to do before we know the final answers? It seems reasonable to suggest that we should follow the prudent course, which would be to reduce salt intake to moderate amounts, to get used to not adding salt at the table, clearly a habit that is easily reversible and is particularly relevant for individuals who have a family history of hypertension. Dr. Langford suggests that individuals with a family history and also hypertensives under treatment should restrict their sodium intake to 70 meq daily, in the belief that modest sodium restriction will enable the treated hypertensive patients to obtain "good blood pressure control with less drug intake and, therefore, less drug side effect" (19).

It is not enough, however, for physicians to tell patients with mild hypertension, that is, with levels of diastolic blood pressure of 90–104 mm Hg, to "watch their salt." These patients are at risk for sequaelae of hypertension and their risk of mortality can be lowered by controlling their blood pressure. They must be *followed* by the physicians. Their pressures must be retaken at appropriate intervals as recommended by the Joint National Committee on Detection, Evaluation, and Treatment of High Blood Pressure (20), and if the preliminary prophylactic measures do not control their blood pressure, then according to the results of the HDFP it is important to treat these individuals pharmacologically to blood pressures below 90 mm Hg. The HDFP, however, did not demonstrate a clear-cut benefit in the younger individuals (those under 50) from vigorous stepped-care treatment, and thus salt restriction among these mild hypertensives should be a first step.

REFERENCES

1. E. Weiss, *Psychosomatic Med.*, **1**, 194 (1939).
2. L. Ambard and E. Beaujard, *Arch. Gen. Med.* **193,** 520 (1904).
3. F. M. Allen, *Med. Clin. N. Am.*, **6,** 475 (1922).
4. W. Kempner, *Am. J. Med.*, **4,** 545 (1948).
5. Veterans Administration Cooperative Study Group on Antihypertensive Agents, *J. Am. Med. Assoc.*, **202,** 116 (1967).
6. Veterans Administration Cooperative Study Group on Antihypertensive Agents, *J. Am. Med. Assoc.*, **213,** 1143 (1970).

7. HDFP Cooperative Group, *Preventive Med.,* **5,** 207 (1976).

8. HDFP Cooperative Group, *J. Am. Med. Assoc.,* **237,** 2385 (1977).

9. HDFP Cooperative Group, *Preventive Med.,* **8,** 2 (1979).

10. HDFP Cooperative Group, *Ann. N. Y. Acad. Sci.,* **304,** 254 (1978).

11. HDFP Cooperative Group, *J. Am. Med. Assoc.,* **242,** 2562 (1979).

12. HDFP Cooperative Group, *J. Am. Med. Assoc.,* **242,** 2572 (1979).

13. G. Pickering, *High Blood Pressure,* 2nd ed., Grune & Stratton, New York, 1968, pp. 394–395.

14. J. Parijs, J. V. Joosens, L. Van der Linden, G. Verstreken, and A. K. P. C. Amery, *Am. Heart J.,* **85,** 23 (1973).

15. T. Morgan, A. Gillies, G. Morgan, W. Adam, M. Wilson, and S. Carney, *Lancet,* **1,** 227 (1978).

16. B. Magnani, E. Ambrosioni, R. Agosta, and F. Racco, *Clin. Sci. Molec. Med.,* **51,** 626s (1976).

17. H. G. Langford, R. L. Watson, and J. G. Thomas, *Trans. Am. Clin. Climatol. Assoc.,* **88,** 32 (1976).

18. S. Wassertheil-Smoller (Chairperson), A. Apostolides, M. Miller, A. Oberman, T. Thom, HDFP Cooperative Group, *J. of Comm. Health,* Issue 5, Winter 1979.

19. H. G. Langford, *Heart & Lung: J. Crit. Care* (St. Louis), **10,** 269 (1981).

20. The 1980 Report of the Joint National Committee on Detection, Evaluation, and Treatment of High Blood Pressure. U.S. Department of Health and Human Services, Public Health Service, National Institutes of Health.

13

Vitamin A Analogs in Skin Disease

DOROTHY B. WINDHORST, M.D.

Hoffmann-La Roche Inc. Nutley, New Jersey

HISTORY

More than two millennia ago ancient Egyptians associated certain foods with the prevention of night blindness. In the early part of the 20th century, Sir F. Gowland Hopkins in England and Elmer V. McCollum in the United States, independently conducting nutrition experiments, discovered that rats failed to grow on lard, but thrived on milk and butter fat. Initially, Hopkins used the term "nutritional accessory factors" for the food constituents essential for growth. In his acceptance speech of the Nobel Prize (1929) he said: ". . . as I learned to understand much later, the diet was doubtless deficient in vitamins A and D."

The first clinical application of vitamin A in modern medicine was in the use of eggs, butter, and milk for the treatment of xerophthalmia and night blindness during World War I when milk and butter were scarce. By 1925, vitamin A was recognized to be important for normal epithelial differentiation, and since the 1930s, dermatologists have used vitamin A in attempts to treat skin diseases.

VITAMIN A FUNCTIONS AND CHEMISTRY

Vitamin A (retinol) has multiple functions, relating to growth, normal vision, reproduction, and the integrity and differentiation of epithelial tissue in the trachea, lungs, salivary glands, urinary bladder, ureter, and gastrointestinal tract, as well as in the skin and its appendages.

191

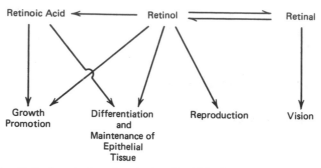

Figure 1.   Retinol, retinal, and retinoic acid—biologic roles and interactions (2).

These biological activities are carried out by three major compounds (1): retinol (vitamin A alcohol), the main dietary source, and the form of its transport and storage; retinal (vitamin A aldehyde), necessary to the formation of rhodopsin, being central to the visual cycle; and retinoic acid, ineffective in the visual cycle and reproduction, but capable of replacing retinol in some of its functions. Retinoic acid has not been found to be stored in the liver, and is therefore thought to be less toxic than retinol.

Figure 1 is a diagrammatic representation of the biological roles of these substances as presented by Pawson (2).

Many newer variations on the structure of retinol have been developed by chemists. These derivatives, as well as retinol, were defined by Sporn (3) as *retinoids*. They were developed initially because of observations that they could affect malignant and premalignant tissues both in vivo and in vitro. As a class of compounds, retinoids have ushered in a new era in the therapy of skin diseases such as cystic acne, psoriasis, and disorders of keratinization notably resistant to other remedies. The structures of some retinoids are shown in Figure 2.

ACTIONS OF RETINOIDS IN MODEL SYSTEMS

In view of an apparent specificity of disease responses to given retinoids—cystic acne to isotretinoin; psoriasis to etretinate—no single theory of mechanism of action can explain all clinical observations. Certainly, a number of poorly understood phenomena are observed when retinoids are added to tissue culture systems. Cultured cells treated with retinoids show profound changes in morphology, such as flattening and increased substrate adhesion, lengthening of generation time, and

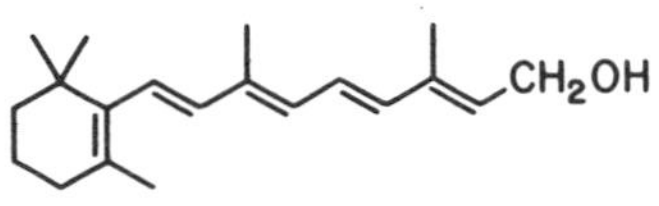

Vitamin A Alcohol, Retinol

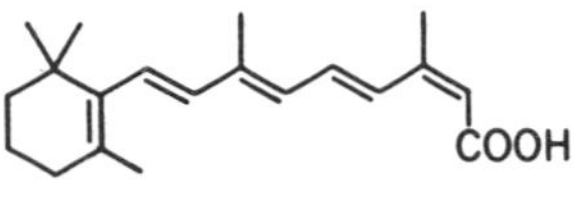

13-*cis*-Retinoic Acid, Isotretinoin

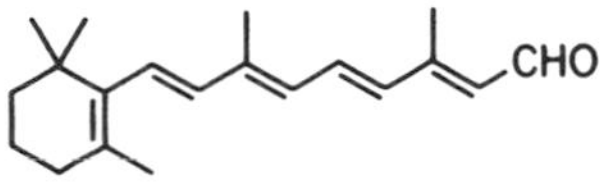

Vitamin A Aldehyde, Retinal

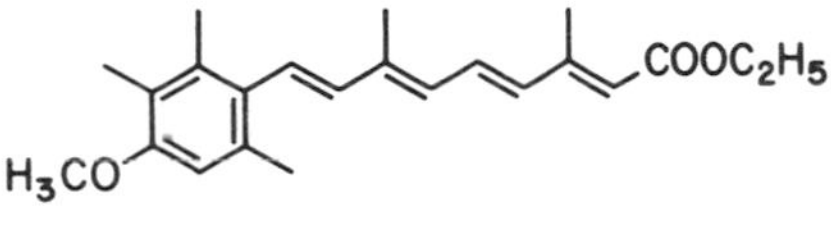

Ro10-9359, Etretinate

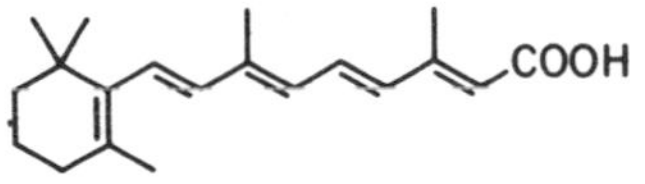

all-*trans* Retinoic Acid, Tretinoin

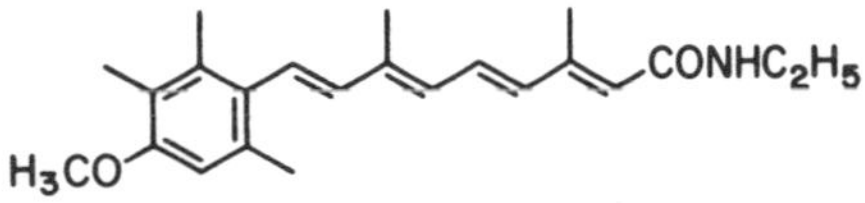

Ro11-1430, Motretinid

Figure 2.   Retinol, retinal, tretinoin, isotretinoin, Ro 10-9359, and Ro 11-1430—chemical structures.

changes in membrane microviscosity, suggesting possible alterations in cell-to-cell interactions.

Effects on Epithelial Tissues

Retinoids promote differentiation toward mucous secretion in epithelial tissues, while inhibiting keratinization and proliferation. In stem cell lines derived from teratocarcinomas the cells differentiate upon exposure to retinoic acid (4). Topically applied, retinoic acid led to regression of carcinogen-induced keratoacanthomas in the rabbit ear (5), an effect accompanied by mucin production and other changes that might be associated with the tumor regression.

Labilization of Membranes

Retinoids appear to act on the lipid bilayers of cell membranes, dramatically decreasing the viscosity of the cell membrane, and destabilizing lysosomes leading to liberation of lysosomal enzymes. On the other hand, at low doses retinoids may stabilize biologic membranes. Faro et al. have presented data on effects in disease states (6).

Effects on the Immune System

Oral retinoids have effects on monocytes, lymphocytes, and related cells. For example, retinoids affected production of arginase in macrophages. The possibility that effects on the immune system may be related to effects of retinoids in cancer has been evaluated by Medawar and Hunt (7).

RETINOIDS AS THERAPY

Initial efforts to treat dermatologic diseases (e.g., psoriasis, the various ichthyoses, and acne) with vitamin A were based on the premise that these disorders reflected a deficiency of intake or proper utilization of the vitamin. Millions of international units (IU) per day were reported in the treatment of psoriasis and mycosis fungoides (8), and in acne vulgaris clinical improvement was described at 300,000 IU/day (9). However, for most dermatological conditions, vitamin A therapy was disappointing, and the newer retinoids developed since the late 1960s have been welcomed as possible alternatives.

The principal aim of the effort to synthesize new analogs of vitamin A was the search for substances that could show a better therapeutic index than retinol or tretinoin in prophylaxis of cancer. Bollag and Matter (10) tested the ability of various retinoids to cause regression of experimentally induced skin lesions in animal models. Sporn et al. (11) screened retinoids for their ability to inhibit keratinization in vitamin A-deficiency-induced squamous metaplasia of tracheal epithelium in organ cultures. These efforts resulted in the synthesis of many new molecules in this group, of which isotretinoin, etretinate, and motretinid have been evaluated in patients with skin disease. As synthetic retinoids have developed, work in Europe focused on etretinate for psoriasis and various congenital ichthyoses, while studies with isotretinoin proceeded in the United States for disorders of keratinization (12) and later for cystic acne.

Psoriasis

The use of vitamin A for psoriasis was never widely accepted, and oral tretinoin was not regarded as very effective in a number of studies over a period of years. The effectiveness of etretinate (ethyl ester of trimethylmethoxyphenyl retinoic acid) given orally to patients with psoriasis was first described by Ott and Bollag (13) in 1975. Numerous other studies have confirmed these results. In a multicenter controlled study, 291 patients given etretinate at initial doses of 70 to 100 mg/day and reduced to 50 mg/day showed significant improvement usually by three weeks. Thereafter, approximately 60% of the patients maintained good or excellent responses on a dose of 25 to 50 mg/day. Scaling, infiltration, and erythema disappeared in that order (14).

Several studies have been suggested that the use of adjunctive therapy enhances the response of plaque psoriasis to etretinate (14, 15) and Fritsch and co-workers (16) observed that etretinate decreased the total amount of ultraviolet radiation needed by psoriatic patients receiving photochemotherapy (methoxsalen and long-wave ultraviolet radiation or PUVA). The combination of retinoid with photochemotherapy has been termed Re-PUVA. It also appeared to be effective in patients who had been PUVA failures previously, including those with palmoplantar psoriasis. One postulated mechanism was that the desquamative effect of etretinate on the psoriatic plaque facilitated the transmission of UVA radiation to the skin.

Cystic Acne

Isotretinoin, 13-*cis*-retinoic acid, is thought to be a metabolite of vitamin A (17). Bollag (18) first published evidence of its usefulness in acne. Furthermore, the early clinical results with psoriasis and leukoplakia by Runne et al. (19) and by Koch and Schettler (20) were a direct consequence of the program for the evaluation of synthetic retinoids developed by Bollag at Hoffmann-La Roche, Basle, Switzerland.

In the study by Peck et al. (21), 13 of 14 patients receiving isotretinoin showed complete clearing of cystic acne with an average maximum dosage of 2.0 mg/kg/day. These patients did not relapse to any significant degree when treatment was stopped after four months, and most patients whose acne had not completely involuted at the end of the treatment period continued to heal after the treatment stopped.

In a second trial reported by Peck et al. (22), isotretinoin was compared to placebo in a parallel randomized double-blind protocol. Doses as low as 0.5 mg/kg/day were effective. Four of 33 patients relapsed and required additional therapy. In a third study, doses of 1.0 to 2.0 mg/kg/day given for only two weeks followed by maintenance doses of 0.25 to 0.5 mg/kg/day appeared to produce comparable therapeutic results.

Plewig et al. (23) confirmed the efficacy of isotretinoin in cystic acne, and explored possible anti-inflammatory effects of the drug. Using the potassium iodide patch test, they found that the intensity of erythema was reduced, along with the number of pustules, within four weeks of beginning treatment. The sebocytes retained nuclei longer than controls, suggesting that isotretinoin alters sebaceous gland differentiation. Etretinate is less effective than isotretinoin both in therapeutic effects on cystic acne and in decreasing sebum production (24), illustrating the differential specificity of the two retinoids.

Since retinoid therapy reduces the size and activity of sebaceous glands and, correspondingly, the sebum production, one effect of isotretinoin in acne may be mediated by an inhibition of sebaceous differentiation. However, sebum production returns toward pretreatment values after discontinuation of therapy, while the acne remains in remission or even improves (22).

Disorders of Keratinization

Both oral and topical retinoic acid (tretinoin) have been used for disorders of keratinization and have been reported to be effective for lamellar ichthyosis, for ichthyosis vulgaris (25), and for palmar and plantar keratoderma (26). European studies have reported that in dosages of 5 to 200 mg/day oral tretinoin was effective in keratosis follicularis, bullous congenital ichthyosiform erythroderma, lichen planus, PRP (pityriasis ruba pilaris), and basal cell epithelioma (27). However, interest in the systemic use of tretinoin declined as isotretinoin and etretinate became available for clinical study.

Numerous reports indicate that Darier's disease, PRP, and lamellar ichthyoses respond to isotretinoin and etretinate. In contrast to its relative lack of effect on cystic acne, etretinate has been reported to produce responses comparable, and possibly superior, to responses produced by isotretinoin in some diseases (28). In diseases that respond to more than one retinoid, the choice will ultimately depend on toxicities of each drug, and on the individual patient's response.

Cancer

Vitamin A deficiency induces a characteristic squamous metaplasia. In the rat this deficiency enhances the susceptibility of the respiratory tract, bladder, and colon to experimental carcinogenesis. Both the changes of vitamin A deficiency and experimental carcinogenesis are reversed by retinoids. Epidemiologic studies have associated the incidence of cancer in humans with decreased serum retinol. The question arises whether increased vitamin A (or β carotene) intake could reduce cancer rates? Attempts to evaluate this question are underway in England and the United States. Patients with multiple basal cell carcinomas, including some with the basal nevus syndrome, were treated with retinoids. In 11 patients, 39 of 248 tumors (16%) underwent complete clinical regression. Examined histologically, more than half of these tumors were considered cured by this criterion. Three patients treated almost continuously for two to four years had no new tumors, while others who discontinued therapy with isotretinoin developed new tumors eight to 18 months after stopping therapy (29). The average maximum dosage was 4.7 mg/kg/day; the maintenance dose averaged 1.5 mg/kg/day.

Variable results have been reported with etretinate in patients with basal cell nevus syndrome, xeroderma pigmentosum, multiple keratoacanthomas, porokeratosis of Mibelli with malignant degeneration, and actinic keratosis (30). New lesions did not occur in a patient with multiple keratoacanthomas when isotretinoin was given continuously after surgical excision of the lesions (31).

TOXICITY OF ORAL RETINOIDS

Toxicity of vitamin A occurs at doses far above the nutritional range, and, in animals, varies with species, dose, and duration of drug administration. In humans, reports of vitamin A toxicity are relatively rare. Between 1850 and 1979, 579 cases of hypervitaminosis A were reported in a total of 195 articles. About 20 of the cases were regarded as severe, none was associated with death, and all appeared to be resolved quickly once the vitamin ingestion was stopped. This is in contrast with an estimated 100,000 individuals reported to be permanently blinded each year and some thousands dead from *lack* of vitamin A (32).

Clinical Toxicity of Retinoids

Toxic effects reported from the systemic use of tretinoin, isotretinoin, and etretinate are similar to those of hypervitaminosis A. Toxicity is dose-dependent in incidence and severity, and reversible on discontinuation of treatment. However, the spectrum of effects varies among compounds, just as the efficacy profile varies across the diseases. Different skin sites are more or less affected by different retinoids.

The most common clinical toxic findings reported for systemic use of the four major retinoids are compared in Table 1, in which the percentages are derived from several articles in the general literature (27, 28, 33). The most interesting aspect of the distribution of signs of retinoid toxicity is the relative prominence of central nervous system symptoms compared to epithelial signs with retinol and tretinoin, and the inverse

Table 1. Stepped Care Treatment Schedule

	Retinol	Tretinoin[a]	Isotretinoln[b]	Etretinate[d]
Integument and mucous membranes				
Cheilitis	37	80	100	100
Inflammation/xerosis	46	50	58	46
Pruritus	34	23	12	12
Thinning of hair	37	1	16	39
Facial dermatitis	—		62	42
Palmoplantar desquamation	—	—	0	47
Paronychia	—	—	0	11
Dryness of mucous membranes	—	30	50	69
Epistaxis, petechiae	—	17	35	46
Eye				
Visual disturbances	37	30	—	—
Bulb pressure increased	—	11	—	—
Conjunctivitis	—	—	77	77
Musculoskeletal				
Bone/joint/muscle complaints	56	—	12	20
Central nervous system				
Headache	40	80	6	Rare
Ataxia	12	—	—	—
Lethargy, fatigue	49	43	0	4
Psychologic changes	27	10	(*)	—
Coma	—	6	—	—
Gastrointestinal				
Anorexia	—	30	—	—
Nausea, vomiting		30	—	—
Weight loss	—	—	—	—
Number of patients		30	26—both drugs	
Average dose (mg/day)		50–200	213	87
Duration of treatment		4 weeks	4–6 months	

[a]Stuttgen (27).
[b]Peck et al. (2).
(*) Meyskens (33).

of this distribution with isotretinoin and etretinate. The latter two compounds also differ as to the efficacy spectrum of areas affected: more facial effects (lips, eyes, dry skin) for isotretinoin, but more palmoplantar effects from etretinate. The latter also has more effects on hair. In the majority of cases the hair loss reported with retinoids is a telogen effluvium; however, dystrophic anagen roots are occasionally found.

All clinical effects are reported to disappear after therapy is discontinued. Studies in growing animals indicate that effects on cartilage and bone are complex, which must be kept in mind if a retinoid is given to a child, as for a congenital ichthyotic condition.

Laboratory Abnormalities

Laboratory abnormalities with retinoid therapy appear to be limited to variable increases in blood lipids, especially triglycerides, in less than one-third of patients, and infrequent abnormalities of liver function tests. Patients who show lipid changes tend to manifest predisposing factors, such as obesity, diabetes, high alcohol intake, or preexisting hyperlipidemia.

Effects on Reproduction

Retinoids at doses higher than used in the clinic may inhibit spermatogenesis in animals, but semen analysis from patients receiving oral retinoids have revealed no abnormalities.

Retinoids are teratogenic when tested in laboratory animals, and the observed minimal teratogenic dose varies between drugs, with etretinate showing effects at lower doses than isotretinoin (34). In fact, some, but not all, fetuses of women who had received etretinate during the first trimester have been abnormal. The slow rate of excretion of etretinate with a consequent long retention in the blood up to 140 days posttreatment restricts its usefulness in females of child-bearing potential. Women receiving any retinoid should use an effective form of contraception.

SUMMARY

Although large doses of oral retinoids produce marked toxic effects in some circumstances, it appears there may be a potential for the use of synthetic retinoids in cancer prevention and therapy in addition to the profoundly important benefits shown thus far in a variety of dermatological conditions. Furthermore, the wide diversity of retinoid effects on cell systems suggests that other, nondermatological, diseases may eventually be found to respond to this new class of therapeutic agents. This is to be expected particularly if newer retinoids show new tissue specificies. As was true of steroids in 1950, the potential of retinoids in 1982 is only partly visible, but very exciting.

REFERENCES

1. H. F. DeLuca et al., "The Metabolism of Retinoic Acid to 5,6-Epoxyretinoic Acid, Retinoyl-B-Glucuronide, and other Polar Metabolites," in L. M. DeLuca and S. S. Shapiro, Eds., *Modulation of Cellular Interaction by Vitamin A and Derivatives (Retinoids)*, New York Academy of Sciences, New York, 1981, p. 25.

2. B. A. Pawson, "A Historical Introduction to the Chemistry of Vitamin A and its Analogs (retinoids)," in L. M. DeLuca and S. S. Shapiro, Eds., *Modulation of Cellular Interaction by Vitamin A and Derivatives (Retinoids)*, New York Academy of Sciences, New York, 1981, p. 1.

3. M. B. Sporn et al., *Fed. Proc.*, **35**, 1332 (1976).

4. M. I. Sherman et al., "Studies on the Mechanism of Induction of Embryonal Carcinoma Cell Differentiation by Retinoic Acid," in L. M. DeLuca and S. S. Shapiro, Eds., *Modulation of Cellular Interaction by Vitamin A and Derivatives (Retinoids)*, New York Academy of Sciences, New York, 1981, p. 192.

5. L. Prutkin, *J. Invest. Dermatol.*, **49**, 165 (1967).

6. R. M. Farb et al., *J. Invest. Dermatol.*, **75**, 133 (1980).

7. P. B. Medawar and R. Hunt, *Immunology*, **42**, 349 (1981).

8. A. Schimpf and K. H. Jansen, *Fortschr. Ther.*, **90**, 635 (1972).

9. A. M. Kligman, J. J. Leyden, and O. Mills, "Oral Vitamin A (retinol) in Acne Vulgaris," in C. E. Orfanos et al., Eds., *Retinoids-Advances in Basic Research and Therapy*, Springer-Verlag, Berlin, 1981, p. 245.

10. W. Bollag and A. Matter, "From Vitamin A to Retinoids in Experimental and Clinical Oncology: Achievements, Failures, and Outlook," in L. M. DeLuca and S. S. Shapiro, Eds., *Modulation of Cellular Interaction by Vitamin A and Derivatives (Retinoids)*, New York Academy of Sciences, New York, 1981, p. 9.

11. M. B. Sporn et al., *Nature*, **263**, 110 (1976).

12. G. L. Peck and F. W. Yoder, *Lancet*, **2**, 1172 (1976).

13. F. Ott and W. Bollag, *Schweiz. Med. Wochenschr.*, **105**, 439 (1975).

14. C. E. Orfanos and G. Goerz, *Dtsch. Med. Wochenschr.*, **103**, 195 (1978).

15. T. Fredriksson, "The Posology of Oral Retinoids: How Much, How Often, How Long?" in C. E. Orfanos et al., Eds., *Retinoids—Advances in Basic Research and Therapy*, Springer-Verlag, Berlin, 1981, p. 349.

16. P. O. Fritsch et al., *J. Invest. Dermatol.*, **70**, 178 (1978).

17. C. A. Frolik, "In vitro and in vivo Metabolism of All-*trans*-and 13-*cis*-Retinoic Acid in the Hamster," in L. M. DeLuca and S. S. Shapiro, Eds., *Modulation of Cellular Interac-*

tion by Vitamin A and Derivatives (Retinoids), New York Academy of Sciences, New York, 1981, p. 37.

18. W. Bollag, Belgian patent 762,344, August 2, 1971.

19. U. Runne et al., *Arch. Dermatol. Forsch.,* **247,** 171 (1973).

20. H. Koch and D. Schettler, *Dtsch. Zahnaerztl. Z.,* **28,** 623 (1973).

21. G. L. Peck et al., *N. Engl. J. Med.,* **300,** 329 (1979).

22. G. L. Peck et al., *J. Am. Acad. Dermatol.,* **6(4),** 735 (1982).

23. G. Plewig et al., "Effects of Two Retinoids in Animal Experiments and After Clinical Application in Acne Patients: 13-*cis*-Retinoic Acid Ro 4-3780 and Aromatic Retinoid Ro 10-9359," in C. E. Orfanos et al., Eds., *Retinoids—Advances in Basic Research and Therapy,* Springer-Verlag, Berlin, 1981, p. 219.

24. J. Goldstein et al., *J. Am. Acad. Dermatol.,* **6(4),** 760 (1982).

25. S. A. Muller et al., *Arch. Dermatol.,* **113,** 1052 (1977).

26. H. B. Heiss and P. R. Gross, *Arch. Dermatol.,* **101,** 100 (1970).

27. G. Stuttgen, *Acta Dermato-Venerologica,* **55(S74),** 174 (1975).

28. G. L. Peck, E. G. Gross, and D. Butkus, "Comparative Analysis of Two Retinoids in the Treatment of Disorders of Keratinization," in C. E. Orfanos et al., Eds., *Retinoids—Advances in Basic Research and Therapy,* Springer-Verlag, Berlin, 1981, p. 279.

29. G. L. Peck, E. G. Gross, D. Butkus, and J. J. DiGiovanna, *J. Am. Acad. Dermatol.,* **6(4),** 815 (1982).

30. L. Schnitzler and J. L. Verret, "Retinoid and Skin Cancer Prevention," in C. E. Orfanos et al., Eds., *Retinoids—Advances in Basic Research and Therapy,* Springer-Verlag, Berlin, 1981, p. 385.

31. R. P. Haydey et al., *N. Engl. J. Med.,* **303,** 560 (1980).

32. J. C. Bauernfeind, *The Safe Use of Vitamin A: A Report on the International Vitamin A Consultative Group (IVAG),* The Nutrition Foundation, Washington, DC, 1980.

33. F. L. Meyskens, *J. Am. Acad. Dermatol.,* **6(4),** 824 (1982).

34. J. J. Kamm, *J. Am. Acad. Dermatol.,* **6(4),** 652 (1982).

Index